DR. JEAN-MICHEL COHEN
FRANCE'S FOREMOST NUTRITION EXPERT

LIGHT
FRENCH RECIPES

A PARISIAN DIET COOKBOOK

Photography by Bernard Radvaner
Photo Styling by Géraldine Sauvage

Flammarion

Acknowledgments

The author wishes to thank the following people for their hard work and their contributions to this book:
Solenne Demanche, Astrid Lorcet, Lucie Picaud, Lucie Marques, and Isabelle Cauët

Translated from the French by Anne McDowall
Design: Alice Leroy
Copyediting: Helen Woodhall
Typesetting: Thierry Renard
Proofreading: Nicole Foster
Indexing: Cambridge Publishing Management Ltd
Color Separation: Jouve Saran, France
Printed in China by Toppan Leefung

Originally published in French as *100 recettes pour alléger nos classiques*
© Flammarion, S.A., Paris, 2010

English-language edition
© Flammarion, S.A., Paris, 2014

editions.flammarion.com

14 15 16   3 2 1

ISBN: 978-2-08-020175-1

Dépôt légal: 04/2014

Contents

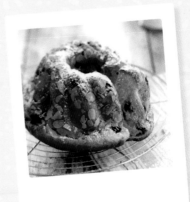

RECIPES

300 CAL/PORTION

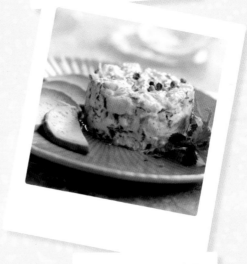

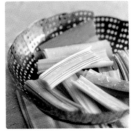

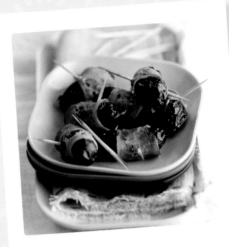

400 CAL/PORTION

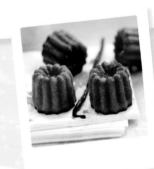

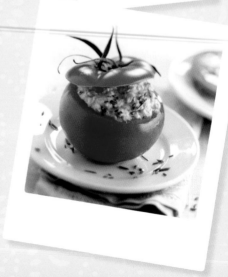

500 CAL/PORTION

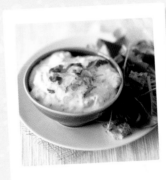

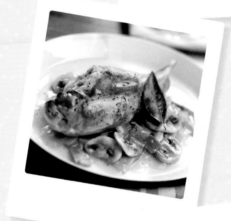

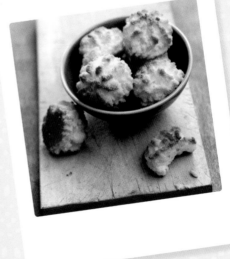

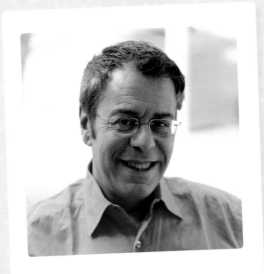

Introduction

You really *can* lose weight *and* enjoy your meals.

It makes me particularly happy when I'm in a consultation and a patient says to me, "I don't understand: I've managed to lose weight while enjoying my food and eating more than I did before." It's not a miracle, it's simply a dieting method I've developed. Weight loss is often linked to deprivation and prohibitions—a diet becomes an "abnormal" period of time that leaves you with bad memories. My desire is to help you reestablish positive eating habits. Let's start talking about foods you *can* eat rather than those you can't!

The way in which you compose a meal or choose a recipe will have an effect on the way you feel throughout the rest of the day. The ratio of proteins, carbohydrates, and fats in your diet will determine whether you feel satisfied, hungry, or have cravings. If the proportions of these nutrients are incorrect, you risk succumbing to afternoon snacking and/or eating more at the next meal to compensate. Instead, if your diet is balanced, with a sufficient intake of fiber, the right amount of fat, and a good proportion of protein, you will attain the winning combination of satiating your hunger, respecting your body, and, if you choose your recipes well, enjoying what you eat.

Boeuf bourguignon, veal blanquette, and other great classics of French cuisine are often regarded as taboo because they're too heavy or high in fat. Yet the flavors and combinations of ingredients in such dishes make them particularly interesting nutritionally, as well as pleasurable to eat. And if you get smart by learning how to measure fat intake and using new cooking methods and light ingredients that you can find in the supermarket, you can easily reduce the calories in classic French dishes without losing out on taste. For example, you can make a light version of cassoulet, a traditional stew from the south of France, by swapping pork sausages for chicken ones, replacing duck confit with lean duck fillet or breast, and adding carrots and tomatoes—rich in antioxidants—to accompany the white (haricot) beans. For dessert, rediscover the pleasure of eating profiteroles: light choux pastry made with cornstarch (cornflour) and light butter, ricotta mixed with applesauce, and a drizzle of dark unsweetened chocolate—that's all there is to it!

These traditional dishes—with their mix of proteins (meat, fish, and dairy products); vegetables, which are indispensable for good health due to the antioxidants they contain; and slow-burning carbohydrates, essential for healthy muscles and brain—have nourished French men and women for generations and give French cuisine its inimitable reputation. They are often complete meals that help you to avoid hunger pangs while providing a balance of ingredients that meets all your nutritional needs. And cooking these dishes will allow you not only to enjoy your food and eat sensibly, but also to join with generations of French people in passing on food-related values that are all too often neglected: family mealtimes, friendly discussions, childhood memories, and the preservation of traditions. A good diet is about respecting the three fundamentals of eating: food should be nutritious, good to share, and pleasurable to eat.

The recipes in this book are divided into three sections, according to the number of calories they contain: 300, 400, or 500 calories maximum per portion. Whether you simply want to eat healthily, stabilize your weight, or shed a few pounds, you'll find yourself delving into these traditional light recipes again and again and will adopt new culinary habits that will benefit and delight the whole family.

These recipes have been created as a way to enjoy the best of French cuisine without guilt, but you can also use them if you are following The Parisian Diet, as part of the Bistro or Gourmet phases. Dieters can turn to pages 8–13 for an overview of the weight-loss program and pages 14–17 for sample daily menus that integrate recipe suggestions from one of the three sections of this book. To learn more about my method, and for nutritional advice and more than 325 recipes, refer to my book *The Parisian Diet: How to Reach Your Right Weight and Stay There* (Flammarion, 2013). To receive two weeks of free access to The Parisian Diet online weight-loss coaching program, go to **http://theparisiandiet.com/promo**.

Jean Michel Cohen

The Parisian Diet: An Overview

Diets that promise quick and easy solutions are alluring, but full of false promises that will keep you from achieving and sustaining your goal. Real success in weight loss can only be achieved by eating a well-balanced diet, based on medical expertise and adapted to modern life. And by doing so intelligently. My method is very simple, you just need some determination to implement it.

With The Parisian Diet, you learn how to rebalance your eating habits. This diet ensures that you take in enough nutrients and—because no food groups are off limits—you won't get frustrated. It's not a revolutionary diet or a trendy one, but a simple process of learning—or relearning—how and what to eat that allows you to achieve a new healthy balance in your life. The practical, realistic guidelines also help you to stay healthy and maintain your new weight after dieting, a challenge that is a common pitfall after following other diets. At its core, The Parisian Diet gives you all the tools you need to achieve a varied and healthy diet (for life!) and one in which pleasure is the key word!

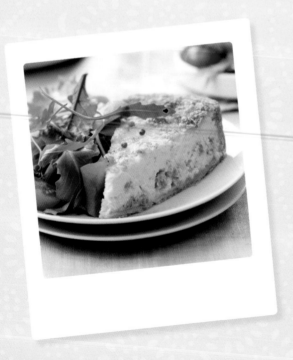

The Parisian Diet offers, rather than imposes (the nuance is important), three phases:

- **Café phase** an optional and brief kick-start where you will lose up to 1 pound (500 g) per day for up to a maximum of ten days
- **Bistro phase** to follow for two to three weeks—you will lose 8 to 11 pounds (3.5–5 kg)
- **Gourmet phase** where you will comfortably lose another 8 to 11 pounds (3.5–5 kg) the first month, followed by an additional 6 to 9 pounds (2.5–4 kg) every month thereafter for at least three months.

The Café phase, designed for healthy adults, allows you to lose the first few pounds in a short time at the beginning of your diet, to give you the incentive to continue. Every pound you lose will give you the motivation to lose the next and help you make the commitment to stick with The Parisian Diet over time. It is optional, intentionally challenging, and short term. This highly restrictive phase of the diet should only be undertaken by people in good health for a loss of up to one pound (400–500 g) per day over a maximum of eight to ten days. Multivitamin and magnesium supplements are obligatory during the Café phase. This phase can also be used for a short period of one to two days for a weight-loss boost of up to one pound (400–500 g) per day if you hit a plateau while following the Bistro or Gourmet phases, or as part of the recovery plan to compensate for the occasional indulgence.

The Café phase includes a lot of liquids: smoothies, purees, soups, and beverages such as water, tea, and black coffee. The nutritional principle is simple: consume a low-calorie diet that is extremely rich in minerals, vitamins, and trace elements. For example, because soups are very filling due to their high micronutrient content, they are effective at counteracting hunger pangs.

The recipes in this book are geared to dieters following the Bistro and Gourmet phases or non-dieters looking for healthy French recipes; information on the Café phase as well as Classic Café menu options can be found in *The Parisian Diet: How to Reach Your Right Weight and Stay There*.

The Bistro phase allows for rapid weight loss of 8 to 11 pounds (3.5–5 kg) in three weeks. It's fast because it's very restrictive. While it will decrease your appetite, it is challenging to maintain over time and is therefore designed for a maximum of three weeks before switching to the Gourmet phase for one month. After that period, you can continue alternating weeks of the Bistro and Gourmet phases until you reach your target weight.

The Bistro phase can also be used for seven days if you hit a weight loss plateau during the Gourmet phase; for two weeks if the Café phase is too difficult to maintain; or for a two to three day treatment if you gain a few pounds after reaching your target weight.

BISTRO PHASE: SAMPLE DAILY ALLOWANCE

Breakfast
- Black coffee, tea, or herbal tea in unlimited quantities, with sweetener and 2 tablespoons (1 fl. oz./30 ml) fat-free milk, if desired.
- ¾ cup (6 oz./175 g) nonfat plain yogurt with sweetener if desired, or 1 cup (8 fl. oz./240 ml) fat-free milk, or equivalent protein.

Lunch
- Raw vegetables or salad in unlimited quantities, seasoned with unsweetened lemon juice, vinegar, mustard, shallots, onions, garlic, herbs, and spices, if desired.
- 3 oz. (85 g) lean meat, fish, or 2 medium eggs, or equivalent protein, cooked without fat.
- Non-starchy vegetables, boiled or steamed without fat, in unlimited quantities.

- ¾ cup (6 oz./175 g) nonfat plain yogurt with sweetener, or 1 cup (8 fl. oz./240 ml) fat-free milk, or equivalent protein.
- 1 piece (5 oz./140 g) of fruit.

Dinner
- Raw vegetables or salad in unlimited quantities, seasoned with unsweetened lemon juice, vinegar, mustard, shallots, onions, garlic, herbs, and spices, if desired.
- 3 oz. (85 g) lean meat, fish, or 2 medium eggs, or equivalent protein, cooked without fat.
- Non-starchy vegetables, boiled or steamed without fat, in unlimited quantities.
- ¾ cup (6 oz./175 g) nonfat plain yogurt with sweetener if desired or 1 cup (8 fl. oz./240 ml) fat-free milk, or equivalent protein.
- 1 piece (5 oz./140 g) of fruit.

The Gourmet phase is designed for pure enjoyment and consists of delicious menus that make it easy to stay on course long term. On average, you can expect to lose 8 to 11 pounds (3.5–5 kg) the first month, and, depending on the individual, 6 to 9 pounds (2.5–4 kg) for each subsequent month. During the Gourmet phase, if your weight loss stagnates, you can follow the Café or Bistro phases for a few days to lose a couple of pounds.

Throughout the Bistro and Gourmet phases, lunch and dinner recipes can be transposed or you can split them to allow you more, but smaller, meals throughout the day, such as a mid-morning or afternoon snack. You may also drink unlimited quantities of black coffee, tea, or herbal tea—with sweetener and 2 tablespoons (1 fl. oz./30 ml) fat-free milk, as desired—between meals, in the morning or afternoon.

GOURMET PHASE: SAMPLE DAILY ALLOWANCE

Breakfast
- Black coffee, tea, or herbal tea in unlimited quantities, with sweetener and 2 tablespoons (1 fl. oz./30 ml) of fat-free milk, if desired.
- 1 slice (1 oz./30 g) bread with 2 level teaspoons (Ð oz./10 g) butter or margarine, or 1 oz. (30 g) unfrosted whole grain breakfast cereal (1 cup light cereal, e.g. cornflakes, or ½ cup heavy cereal, e.g. wheat bran, less than 380 calories per 3 ½ oz./100 g) and 6 nuts (e.g. almonds, walnuts, cashews).
- ¾ cup (6 oz./175 g) plain nonfat yogurt, with sweetener if desired, or equivalent protein.
- 1 piece (5 oz./140 g) of fruit.

Lunch
- Raw vegetables or salad in unlimited quantities seasoned with 1 teaspoon oil and unlimited lemon juice, vinegar, mustard, shallots, onion, herbs.
- 4 oz. (115 g) lean meat, cooked without fat, or equivalent protein.

- Vegetables boiled or steamed without fat, in unlimited quantities.
- ¾ cup (6 oz./175 g) plain nonfat yogurt with sweetener if desired or equivalent protein.
- 1 piece (5 oz./140 g) of fruit.

Dinner
- Raw vegetables or salad in unlimited quantities seasoned with 1 teaspoon oil and unlimited lemon juice, vinegar, mustard, shallots, onion, herbs, or vegetable soup (max. 100 calories and 3.5 g fat per serving).
- 4 oz. (115 g) lean meat, cooked without fat, or equivalent protein.
- 3 ½ oz. (100 g) cooked carbohydrates (pasta, rice, couscous, potato) or 1 oz. (30 g) dried (pasta, rice, couscous) with 1 level teaspoon (¼ oz./7 g) butter or margarine.
- Vegetables, boiled or steamed without fat, in unlimited quantities.
- 1 oz. (30 g) cheese (less than 50% milk fat), or equivalent protein.
- 1 piece (5 oz./140 g) of fruit.

Food Equivalents and Substitutes

The following list of food alternatives can be used to add variety to the recipes, or to replace a food you don't particularly enjoy or that is not readily available or in season.

Protein (meat, fish, poultry, cheese)

4 oz. (115 g) cooked chicken or turkey (white meat, no skin)

2 medium eggs

4 oz. (115 g) cooked fish fillet (cod, flounder, haddock, halibut, salmon, trout, tuna—fresh, frozen, or canned in brine)

4 oz. (115 g) shellfish, cleaned and shells removed (clams, crab, lobster, scallops, shrimp)

3 oz. (85 g) lean ham, not marbled

4 oz. (115 g) cooked lean meat: lean beef trimmed of fat (round/topside, sirloin, flank steak); beef tenderloin/fillet; roast beef (chuck, rib); steak (T-bone, porterhouse, cubed); ground round/lean minced beef (10–15% fat); cooked lean pork; pork tenderloin; center pork loin chop; lean lamb chop; veal

4 oz. (115 g) firm tofu

2 oz. (55 g) hard cheese (cheddar, mozzarella, Swiss, Parmesan, American)

1 ½ cups (12 oz./340 g) plain nonfat yogurt

1 cup (8 oz./225 g) 2% milk fat cottage cheese

⅓ cup (6 oz./175 g) 4% milk fat cottage cheese

Vegetables

2 cups (8 oz./225 g) diced cucumber

2 cups (10 oz./280 g) raw leafy greens (salad greens, sauerkraut, spinach)

1 cup (6 oz./175 g) cooked leafy greens (Brussels sprouts, cabbage, celery, leeks, scallions [spring onions])

1 cup (6 oz./175 g) cooked vegetables (artichoke, asparagus, broccoli, cauliflower, eggplant [aubergine], mushroom, pepper, pumpkin, radish, tomato)

½ cup (3 oz./85 g) cooked diced starchy vegetables (yam, potato, sweet potato, green peas, plantain)

½ cup (3 oz./85 g) cooked beans, lentils, peas (chickpeas, black-eyed peas, pinto beans, kidney beans)

Carbohydrates/Starches

2 ½ tablespoons (1 oz./30 g) uncooked rice

½ cup (3 ½ oz./100 g) cooked rice

⅓ cup (1 ½ oz./40 g) raw pasta

¾ cup (3 ½ oz./100 g) cooked pasta

½ bagel

1 slice (1 oz./30 g) bread

½ pita bread (6-in./15-cm diameter)

2 tablespoons (1 oz./30 g) dry oats

½ cup (3 oz./85 g) cooked whole oats

Milk and Dairy Products

½ cup (4 fl. oz./120 ml) 1% or 2% milk

1 cup (8 fl. oz./240 ml) fat-free milk

2 level tablespoons (½ oz./15 g)
powdered milk

¾ cup (6 oz./175 g) plain low-fat yogurt

1 cup (8 oz./225 g) plain nonfat yogurt

1 oz. (30 g) hard cheese (American, cheddar,
mozzarella, Parmesan, Swiss)

¼ cup (2 oz./55 g) whole milk ricotta cheese

⅓ cup (3 oz./85 g) part-skim ricotta cheese

⅓ cup (3 oz./85 g) 4% milk fat cottage cheese

½ cup (4 oz./115 g) 2% milk fat cottage cheese

⅓ cup (5 oz./140 g) 1% milk fat cottage cheese

Fats

1 strip bacon

1 tablespoon (½ oz./15 g) nonfat cream
cheese, sandwich spread, or sour cream

1 teaspoon (¼ oz./7 g) butter or margarine
or vegetable oil

2 teaspoons (⅓ oz./10 g) mayonnaise
or peanut butter

6 nuts (almonds, cashews)

10 peanuts

10 olives

Fruit

1 small fruit / 1 slice / 1 cup (5 oz./140 g)
(chopped) any fruit

1 ½ tablespoons (½ oz./15 g) raisins

8 halves dried apricots

1 ½ dried figs

3 whole dates, pitted

3 prunes, dried, pitted

100% fruit juice:

½ cup (4 fl. oz./120 ml) apple juice

⅓ cup (2 ¾ fl. oz./80 ml) cranberry juice

1 cup (8 fl. oz./240 ml) cranberry juice
(lite or reduced calorie)

⅓ cup (2 ¾ fl. oz./80 ml) grape juice

½ cup (4 fl. oz./120 ml) grapefruit juice

½ cup (4 fl. oz./120 ml) orange juice

½ cup (4 fl. oz./120 ml) pineapple juice

⅓ cup (2 ¾ fl. oz./80 ml) prune juice

Wine

Parisians enjoy wine—either as an aperitif
before a meal or a glass with a meal.
A small (4 ¼ fl. oz./125 ml) glass can
be substituted for a serving of fruit.

Sample Menus

The following sample menus provide menu options for readers wishing to follow the Bistro and Gourmet phases of The Parisian Diet. The daily menus can be used in any order you wish. Different menus can be swapped around or repeated as desired. And for further customization, you can follow the suggestion in the menu for each meal, or choose an option from the sample daily allowance (see pp. 10–11). In addition, each daily menu allows you to choose one of the recipes from the three sections of this book, organized according to the maximum number of calories per portion: for the recipes at 300 Cal/portion, see pp. 20–69; at 400 Cal/portion, see pp. 70–121; and at 500 Cal/portion, see pp. 122–189.

As long as you consume all of the items (or their equivalents) in one full menu each day and you respect the number of calories in the recipe option proposed, you can feel free to invert mealtimes, having dinner for lunch and vice versa, or replace a main course recipe with a starter recipe within the same section, if you so desire. The most important thing to keep in mind when customizing the following menus is to stay faithful to the given quantities, because it's the balance between the portions and food groups that makes the difference between a healthy diet and one that is too rich.

Bistro Phase

BISTRO MENU 1

Breakfast	Lunch	Dinner
Black coffee, tea, or herbal tea	3 oz. (80 g) lean roast beef	Choose one main course
¾ cup (6 oz./175 g) plain nonfat yogurt, with sweetener if desired	6 oz. (175 g) broccoli, steamed with nutmeg	recipe at **500 Cal/ portion**
	1 kiwi	1 orange

BISTRO MENU 2

Breakfast	Lunch	Dinner
Black coffee, tea, or herbal tea	Choose one starter or main course recipe at **300 Cal/ portion**	3 oz. (80 g) turkey breast, grilled without fat, with lemon juice and thyme
1 slice (1 oz./30 g) wholegrain bread, toasted	½ grapefruit	6 oz. (175 g) finely sliced zucchini (courgette), stir-fried without fat
2 teaspoons (⅓ oz./8.5 g) peanut butter		1 kiwi
¾ cup (6 oz./175 g) plain nonfat yogurt, with sweetener if desired		
½ grapefruit		

BISTRO MENU 3

Breakfast
Black coffee, tea, or herbal tea
1 slice (1 oz./30 g) wholegrain bread
1 medium egg, dry-fried
½ cup (4 oz./115 g) 1% milk fat cottage cheese

Lunch
3 oz. (80 g) cod fillet, oven-baked with parsley
6 oz. (175 g) roasted tomatoes, with garlic and fresh chopped basil
⅓ cup (3 oz./80 g) plain nonfat yogurt, with sweetener if desired

Dinner
Choose one starter or main course recipe at **300 Cal/ portion**
½ cup (3 ½ oz./100 g) fresh pineapple chunks

BISTRO MENU 4

Breakfast
Black coffee, tea, or herbal tea
¾ cup (6 oz./175 g) plain nonfat yogurt, with sweetener if desired
1 apple

Lunch
Choose one starter or main course recipe at **400 Cal/ portion**
⅓ cup (3 oz./80 g) plain nonfat yogurt, with a few drops of vanilla extract if desired

Dinner
Salad comprised of: 2 cups (4 oz./ 115 g) shredded red cabbage
1 medium egg, hard-boiled and sliced
½ cup (4 oz./115 g) 1% milk fat cottage cheese
1 ½ tablespoons (½ oz./15 g) raisins
Lemon juice to season

BISTRO MENU 5

Breakfast
Black coffee, tea, or herbal tea
1 slice (1 oz./30 g) wholegrain bread
½ cup (4 oz./115 g) 1% milk fat cottage cheese
2 oz. (60 g) lean ham

Lunch
2 oz. (60 g) firm tofu, stir-fried without fat, with soy sauce
6 oz. (175 g) diced eggplant (aubergine), dry-fried with basil
½ cup (4 oz./115 g) plain nonfat yogurt

Dinner
Choose one starter or main course recipe at **400 Cal/ portion**
½ cup (4 oz./115 g) plain nonfat yogurt, with a few drops of vanilla extract if desired

BISTRO MENU 6

Breakfast
Black coffee, tea, or herbal tea
Choose one dessert recipe at **300 Cal/portion**

Lunch
Omelet made with 2 eggs and basil, cooked without fat
½ cup (¾ oz./20 g) arugula
¾ cup (3 oz./80 g) grated raw beet (beetroot)
Balsamic vinegar to season

Dinner
Choose one starter or main course recipe at **300 Cal/ portion**
1 cup (7 oz./200 g) stewed fruit, with no added sugar

BISTRO MENU 7

Breakfast
Black coffee, tea, or herbal tea
½ cup (4 oz./115 g) 1% milk fat cottage cheese

Lunch
4 oz. (115 g) shrimp, dry-fried, with garlic and parsley
6 oz. (175 g) green beans, steamed
Choose one dessert recipe at **300 Cal/portion**

Dinner
1 cup (8 fl. oz./250 ml) vegetable soup, without fat or carbohydrates
2 oz. (60 g) lean chicken ham
¾ cup (6 oz./175 g) plain nonfat yogurt

Gourmet Phase

GOURMET MENU 1

Breakfast
Black coffee, tea, or herbal tea
1 slice (1 oz./30 g) wholegrain
  bread
2 teaspoons (⅓ oz./10 g) regular
  butter
¾ cup (6 oz./175 g) plain nonfat
  yogurt
1 apple

Lunch
1 cup (8 fl. oz./250 ml) vegetable
  soup, with 1 teaspoon oil
4 oz. (115 g) cod fillet, steamed
  with tarragon
7 oz. (200 g) leeks, steamed or
  stewed without fat
½ cup (4 oz./115 g) 1% milk fat
  cottage cheese
4 oz. (115 g) grapes

Dinner
Choose one starter or main
  course recipe at **500 Cal/
  portion**
1 oz. (30 g) cheddar cheese

GOURMET MENU 2

Breakfast
Black coffee, tea, or herbal tea
½ (1 oz./30 g) wholegrain bagel
2 teaspoons (⅓ oz./10 g) peanut
  butter
½ cup (4 oz./115 g) 1% milk fat
  cottage cheese
1 pear

Lunch
Choose one starter or dessert
  recipe at **300 Cal/portion**
4 oz. (115 g) chicken breast,
  dry-fried with curry powder
7 oz. (200 g) green beans,
  steamed

Dinner
2 cups (5 oz./150 g) raw grated
  carrot
1 serving vinaigrette*
4 oz. (115 g) hake, steamed with dill
½ cup (3 ½ oz./100 g) cooked pasta
¾ cup (6 oz./175 g) nonfat plain
  yogurt
1 kiwi

GOURMET MENU 3

Breakfast
Black coffee, tea, or herbal tea
1 large slice (1 oz./30 g) baguette
  (French stick)
2 teaspoons (⅓ oz./10 g) regular
  butter
4 tablespoons (2 oz./60 g) part-
  skim ricotta cheese
½ banana

Lunch
Salad leaves
1 serving vinaigrette*
4 oz. (115 g) rump steak, grilled
7 oz. (200 g) zucchini (courgette),
  dry-fried
¾ cup (6 oz./175 g) nonfat plain
  yogurt
1 apple

Dinner
1 cup (8 fl. oz./250 ml) vegetable
  soup
4 oz. (115 g) extra lean ham
Choose one dessert recipe at
  300 Cal/portion

* Vinaigrette, made with 2 tbs oil, 1 tbs mustard, 3 tbs water, salt and pepper: makes 4 servings

GOURMET MENU 4

Breakfast
Black coffee, tea, or herbal tea
1 slice (1 oz./30 g) wholegrain
  bread
2 teaspoons (⅓ oz./10 g) peanut
  butter
1 oz. (30 g) hard cheese
½ banana

Lunch
2 cups (5 oz./150 g) sliced raw
  tomatoes
1 serving vinaigrette*
4 oz. (115 g) turkey breast,
  cooked without fat
7 oz. (200 g) frozen spinach,
  steamed or stewed without
  fat

¾ cup (6 oz./175 g) nonfat plain
  yogurt
1 pear

Dinner
Choose one starter or main
  course recipe at **500 Cal/portion**
½ cup (4 oz./115 g) 1% milk fat
  cottage cheese

GOURMET MENU 5

Breakfast
Black coffee, tea, or herbal tea
½ (1 oz./30 g) wholegrain bagel
2 teaspoons (⅓ oz./10 g) regular
  butter
¾ cup (6 oz./175 g) plain nonfat
  yogurt
1 orange

Lunch
Choose one starter or main
  course recipe at **400 Cal/portion**
7 oz. (200 g) broccoli, steamed
1 kiwi

Dinner
2 cups (5 oz./150 g) sliced raw
  cucumber, with 1 teaspoon oil
4 oz. (115 g) steak, grilled
½ cup (3 ½ oz./100 g) cooked
  bulgur wheat
½ cup (4 oz./115 g) 1% milk fat
  cottage cheese
1 pear

GOURMET MENU 6

Breakfast
Black coffee, tea, or herbal tea
1 large slice (1 oz./30 g) baguette
  (French stick)
2 teaspoons (⅓ oz./10 g) peanut
  butter
½ cup (4 oz./115 g) 1% milk fat
  cottage cheese
1 kiwi

Lunch
Salad leaves
1 serving vinaigrette*
4 oz. (115 g) chicken wings, grilled
7 oz. (200 g) eggplant (aubergine),
  dry-fried or grilled
¾ cup (6 oz./175 g) nonfat plain
  yogurt
1 apple

Dinner
1 cup (8 fl. oz./250 ml) vegetable
  soup
4 oz. (115 g) turkey breast, dry-
  fried with tandoori spice
Choose one dessert recipe at
  300 Cal/portion

GOURMET MENU 7

Breakfast
Black coffee, tea, or herbal tea
1 oz. (30 g) unfrosted wholegrain
  cereal (1 cup light cereal, e.g.
  cornflakes, or ½ cup heavy
  cereal, e.g. wheat bran) + 1 cup
  (8 fl. oz./250 ml) fat-free milk
10 roasted peanuts
1 grapefruit

Lunch
2 cups (5 oz./150 g) grated raw
  celeriac
1 serving vinaigrette*
4 oz. (115 g) salmon, steamed
  with dill
7 oz. (200 g) carrots, steamed
  or cooked without fat
1 oz. (30 g) cheddar cheese
4 oz. (115 g) grapes

Dinner
Choose one starter or main
  course recipe at **500 Cal/portion**
¾ cup (6 oz./175 g) nonfat plain
  yogurt

10 Tips for Cooking Light

1 Reduce your fat intake by limiting your use of cooking fat and equipping yourself with new kitchen utensils and accessories (nonstick pans, parchment/greaseproof paper to line molds, silicone molds, etc.); by using light fats (light butter, oil sprays, etc.); and by adopting "light" cooking methods (microwaving, steaming, pressure-cooking).

2 Say goodbye to sauces? Sauces are often high in fat because butter or oil is used to emulsify the tasty juices, but it's easy to reduce their fat content. Use skimmed vegetable, chicken, beef, or fish stock. You can choose the intensity of flavor by reducing them to your taste.

3 There are now all sorts of liquid and powder sweeteners available, some of which are suitable for cooking. You can use them to replace sugar in any form.

4 Choose lean cuts of meat to reduce the calorie count of a recipe. Using lean Canadian (back) bacon rather than streaky bacon, for example, will reduce the calorie count by more than half. Make sure you remove all visible fat from pieces of meat.

5 Opt for carbohydrates! Cornstarch (cornflour) and potato starch are very useful for thickening gravies and sauces. In particular, you can use them to lighten béchamel and other sauces, crèmes anglaises, and crèmes pâtissières, or even to replace some of the flour in pastry dishes.

6 Make the most of herbs and spices: as well as enabling you to reduce the quantity of sauce needed to give flavor to dishes, they contain beneficial antioxidants and provide new tastes.

7 Replace full-fat dairy products (cheese, milk, cream) with light versions.

8 Fill your kitchen cupboards with food that you actually need rather than with impulse buys. Keep a list of indispensable food items and take it with you when you go shopping.

9 Cook only the quantity you need and stick to precise portion sizes. This will enable you both to avoid waste and to control your food intake. To get a sense of portion sizes, use tablespoons, glasses, bowls, etc.

10 Serve seasonings separately so that each person can decide how much to take according to their taste.

Recipes

The following classic French favorites
have been adapted and tested by
nutritionists to provide healthy and
delicious alternatives perfect for dieters
and non-dieters alike. They are organized
into three sections by caloric value.

Prunes wrapped in bacon
Pruneaux en robe de filet de bacon

This classic hors d'oeuvre for festive meals is offered here in a light version, simply by replacing streaky bacon with smoked Canadian (back) bacon, which is much lower in fat. A good saving in calories and it tastes nicer too—try it and see if you don't prefer it!

PREP TIME 10 minutes | **COOK TIME** 15 minutes | **REST TIME** 5 minutes

INGREDIENTS FOR 4 PEOPLE
8 slices of extra-lean Canadian-style (back) bacon
16 pitted prunes

1 Preheat the oven to 350°F (180°C/Gas mark 4).

2 Cut the bacon slices in half.

3 Roll each prune in a half slice of bacon and secure with a toothpick (cocktail stick).

4 Arrange on a baking sheet covered with parchment (greaseproof) paper and cook in the oven for about 15 minutes, until the bacon is crispy. Remove from the oven and let stand for 5 minutes before serving.

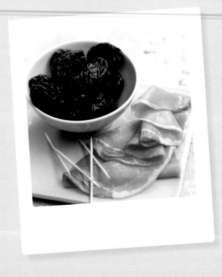

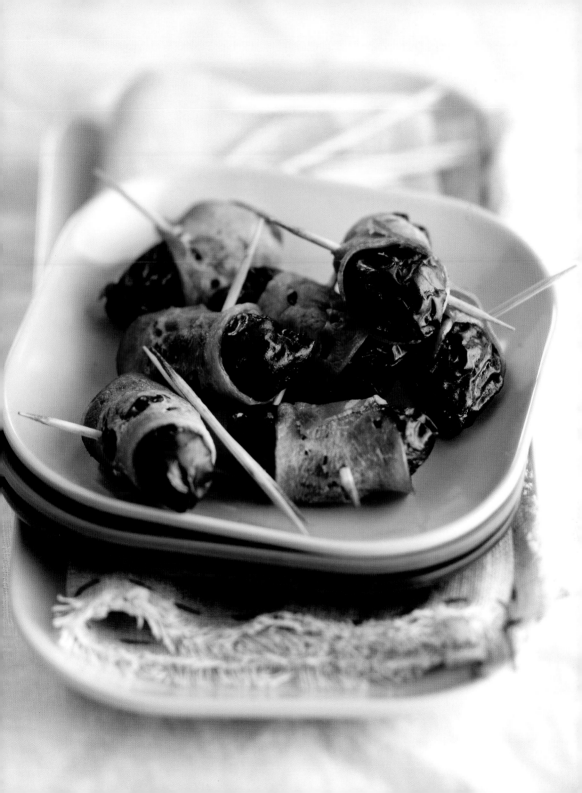

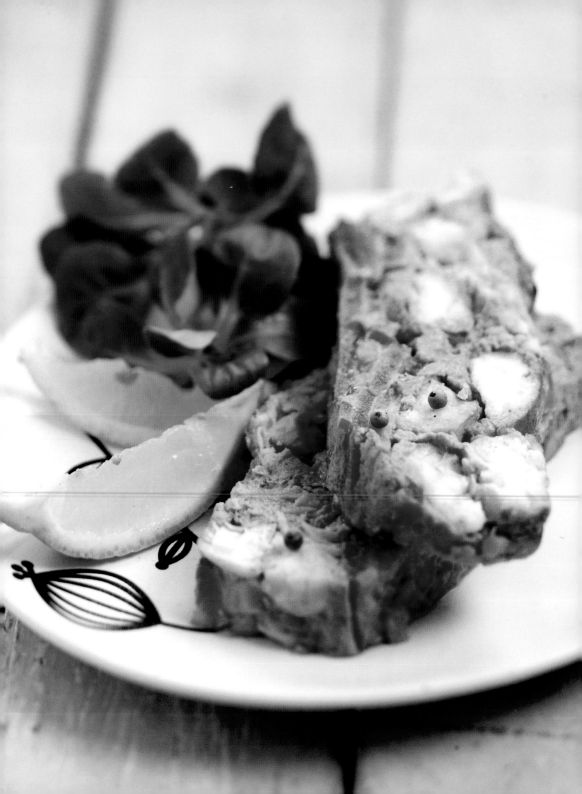

Monkfish terrine on a bed of corn salad

Terrine de lotte sur lit de mâche

Monkfish (anglerfish) is a fine food and a lean fish. Commercial terrines often contain a significant amount of fat, which makes them deceptively calorific. With this quick-and-easy recipe, you'll be able to enjoy a truly light dish.

PREP TIME 35 minutes | **COOK TIME** 55 minutes

INGREDIENTS FOR 4 PEOPLE
4 pints (2 liters) fish stock
Juice of 1 lemon
1 ¾ lb. (800 g) monkfish (anglerfish)
2 eggs
1 ¼ cups (10 fl. oz./300 ml) low-fat sour cream (crème fraîche)
½ teaspoon mild chili powder
½ teaspoon paprika
1 small can tomato paste (purée)
2 tomatoes
7 oz. (200 g) corn salad (lamb's lettuce)
Salt and pepper

1 Preheat the oven to 300°F (150°C/Gas mark 2).

2 Pour the fish stock into a large cooking pot, and add the lemon juice. Add the fish, and cook at a simmer for about 15 minutes to parcook the fish. Beat the eggs with the cream, salt, pepper, spices, and the tomato paste in a bowl.

3 Drain the fish, remove the backbone, and cut into pieces. Wash and slice the tomatoes.

4 Line a small terrine dish with parchment (greaseproof) paper and layer the tomato slices in the bottom, then add the monkfish pieces and pour over the beaten eggs and cream. Cook in the oven for 40 minutes. Serve, still warm and cut in slices, on a bed of corn salad.

Salade niçoise

Salade niçoise is often, rather untraditionally, served with rice in restaurants. This is an authentic recipe for this tasty salad.

PREP TIME 25 minutes

INGREDIENTS FOR 4 PEOPLE
7 oz. (200 g) lettuce
2 or 3 medium (10 oz./280 g) tomatoes
2 medium (10 oz./280 g) red bell peppers
1 can artichoke hearts in water
2 eggs
12 black olives
12 anchovy fillets (not in oil), desalted
1 onion
1 ½ cups (12 oz./320 g) flaked canned tuna in water or brine, drained
2 tablespoons olive oil
4 tablespoons balsamic vinegar
Pinch of herbes de Provence
Salt and pepper

1 Wash the vegetables and drain the artichoke hearts. Hard-boil the eggs. Shred the lettuce and cut the tomatoes, hard-boiled eggs, and artichoke hearts into quarters.

2 Dice the peppers, pit and slice the olives, and chop the anchovies and onion. Drain and flake the tuna.

3 Arrange the lettuce, tomatoes, peppers, and artichoke hearts on a plate, and top with the flaked tuna, hard-boiled egg quarters, and chopped anchovies. Sprinkle over the sliced olives and chopped onion. Season with salt and pepper, and sprinkle with the olive oil, balsamic vinegar, and herbes de Provence.

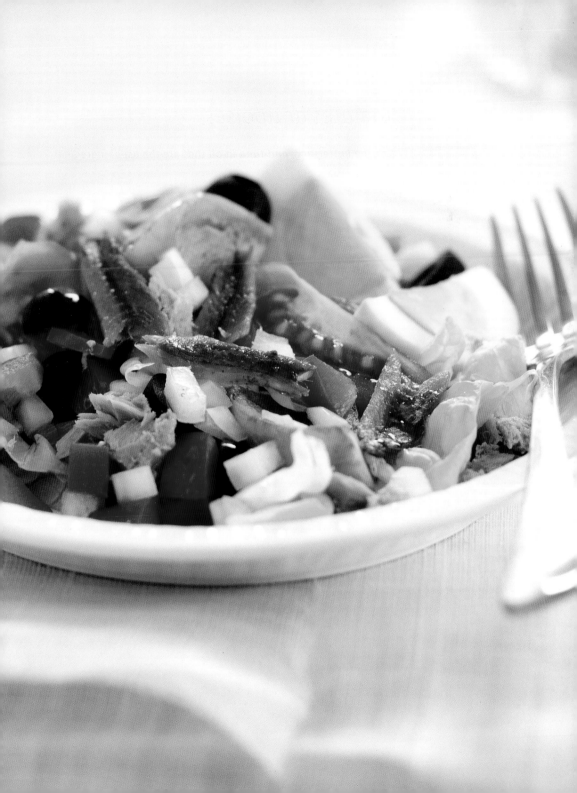

Toasted goat cheese on artichoke hearts
Toasts chèvre-artichaut

Cheese lovers are often partial to delicious warm goat cheese melting on toast. There's no need to banish cheese altogether when you're watching your weight as long as you consume it in moderation. With this recipe, you'll save calories and discover an original food combination by replacing the slice of toast with an artichoke heart.

PREP TIME 10 minutes | **COOK TIME** 20 minutes

INGREDIENTS FOR 4 PEOPLE
4 frozen artichoke hearts
4 cabécous (small round goat cheeses,
    about 1 ¼–1 ½ oz./35–40 g each
    and 1 ½–2 ½ in./4–6 cm diameter;
    if unavailable, substitute another
    round goat cheese, or 4 slices
    of a log-shaped goat cheese)
Pinch of herbes de Provence
Freshly ground pepper
Mixed salad leaves, to serve

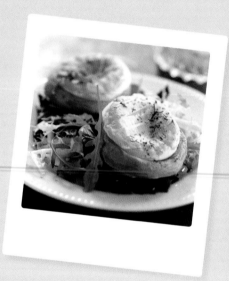

1 Steam cook the artichoke hearts, according to package instructions, until tender.

2 Preheat the oven broiler (grill).

3 Lay the artichoke hearts in an ovenproof dish lined with parchment (greaseproof) paper. Grind over some pepper, top each artichoke heart with a goat cheese, and sprinkle over some herbes de Provence. Place under the broiler (grill) to lightly melt the cheese.

4 Serve on a bed of mixed salad leaves.

Antibes-style tomatoes
Tomates antiboises

Exit the butter, egg, and tuna in oil that are the usual ingredients for this dish. Enter tuna canned in water or brine and a sauce made from nonfat fromage blanc or fat-free cream cheese. So, enjoy this light appetizer guilt-free and benefit from the high omega-3 fatty acid content of the tuna.

PREP TIME 20 minutes | **CHILL TIME** 15 minutes

INGREDIENTS FOR 4 PEOPLE
4 tomatoes (about 14 oz./400 g)
Generous ½ cup (4 ¼ oz./120 g) canned tuna
   in water or brine
⅓ cup (3 oz./80 g) nonfat fromage blanc
   or plain nonfat regular or Greek yogurt
4 teaspoons mustard
4 teaspoons snipped chives
   + some for garnish
Salt and pepper

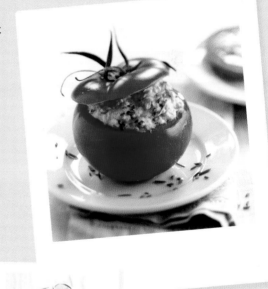

1 Wash the tomatoes and slice off the tops to make lids, then scoop out the flesh. In a bowl, flake the tuna and mix with the tomato flesh. Add the fromage blanc or yogurt, mustard, and chives and mix well. Season to taste.

2 Fill the tomatoes with this mixture, replace their "lids" and refrigerate until required.

3 Before serving, garnish with a few snipped chives.

Snails in garlic and parsley cream

*Petites cassolettes d'escargots
à la crème d'ail et persil*

A dozen snails are a favorite first course at festive meals in France, but it's usually a high-calorie choice. In fact, snails are very lean; it's the butter they're served with that makes the calorie count rocket! This dish is made with low-fat thick (light double) cream, which is much lower in fat than butter so you can enjoy this pleasure while dieting.

PREP TIME 15 minutes | **COOK TIME** 30 minutes

INGREDIENTS FOR 4 PEOPLE
2 cloves garlic
14 oz. (400 g) snails
½ bunch parsley
4 tablespoons low-fat sour cream (crème fraîche)
Salt and pepper

1 Preheat the oven to 350°F (180°C/Gas mark 4).

2 Peel and finely chop the garlic. Dry-fry in a nonstick skillet (frying pan) until golden. Add the snails and cook for an additional 10 minutes over a medium heat.

3 Divide the snails between four individual ovenproof dishes.

4 Mix the parsley with the cream in a blender or food processor. Season with salt and pepper. Pour over the snails and cook in the oven for 15 minutes.

5 Serve hot.

Salade landaise

Specialties of the Landes in southwest France often include duck confit, foie gras, and lots of calories. Even though it's a salad, the famous salade landaise *can be heavy. This delicious recipe marries preserved duck gizzards, baby spinach leaves, and a moderate amount of tasty dressing containing walnut oil. The reduction in calories will not reduce the taste of this gourmet dish.*

PREP TIME 20 minutes | **COOK TIME** 10 minutes

INGREDIENTS FOR 4 PEOPLE
10 ½ oz. (300 g) baby spinach leaves
10 ½ oz. (300 g) purslane
10 ½ oz. (300 g) preserved duck gizzards
   (if unavailable, substitute chicken livers)
1 tablespoon wine vinegar
2 tablespoons walnut oil
1 bunch chervil
Salt and pepper

1   Wash, trim, and dry the baby spinach leaves and purslane.

2   Rinse the duck gizzards under hot running water to remove the fat that's coating them. Dry them on absorbent paper towels. Dry-fry them in a nonstick skillet (frying pan) over a low heat for a minute until browned.

3   In a salad bowl, make the dressing by mixing together salt, pepper, and the vinegar, then the walnut oil.

4   Tip the baby spinach leaves, purslane, and chervil leaves into the salad bowl and toss well to coat in the dressing. Put the warm duck gizzards on top before serving.

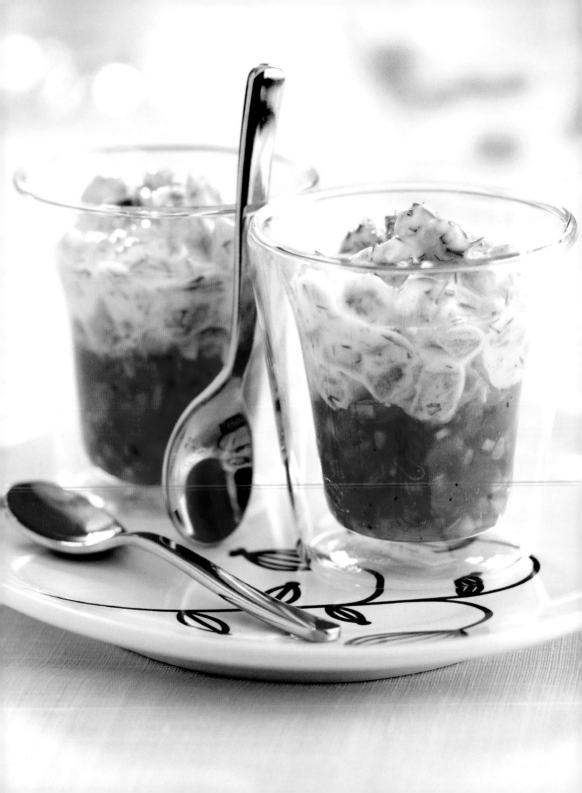

Salmon and dill verrines
Verrines de saumon à l'aneth

Salmon tartare served in restaurants is often covered in a thick layer of oil, but this recipe, made with only two teaspoons of oil, is light and refreshing, and is served in pretty glasses to add elegance to your table.

PREP TIME 30 minutes | **CHILL TIME** 25 minutes

INGREDIENTS FOR 4 PEOPLE
7 oz. (200 g) very fresh salmon fillet
1 lime
2 shallots
3 tomatoes
½ bunch dill
4 tablespoons (2 oz./60 g) nonfat fromage blanc
　　or plain nonfat regular or Greek yogurt
2 teaspoons olive oil
Salt and pepper

1　Finely dice the salmon and set aside in the refrigerator.

2　Squeeze the juice from the lime and peel and finely chop the shallots. Immerse the tomatoes in boiling water for a few seconds to loosen their skins, then peel and dice. Chop the dill reserving a few sprigs for decoration.

3　In a bowl, mix the fromage blanc or yogurt, lime juice, chopped dill, salt, and pepper. Stir this sauce into the diced salmon.

4　In another bowl, mix the diced tomatoes, shallots, and olive oil and season to taste with salt and pepper.

5　Divide the tomato and shallot mixture between four small glasses, then cover with the salmon and fromage blanc or yogurt mixture. Refrigerate until ready to serve.

6　Decorate with sprigs of dill before serving.

Artichokes with brocciu cheese
Artichauts au brocciu

Why not take advantage of this fabulous, particularly low-fat fresh Corsican cheese to serve artichokes in a different way, rather than dipping the leaves in an often calorie-laden mayonnaise or vinaigrette?

PREP TIME 45 minutes | **COOK TIME** 1 hour 10 minutes

INGREDIENTS FOR 4 PEOPLE

7 oz. (200 g) brocciu cheese (if unavailable, substitute another low-fat fresh goat or ewe's milk cheese)

4 tomatoes

2 onions

1 clove garlic

1 sprig thyme

1 sprig rosemary

3 ½ oz. (100 g) lean smoked Canadian-style (back) bacon

1 egg

8 small (young) artichokes

½ lemon

2 crispbreads

Salt and pepper

1 Drain the brocciu.

2 Immerse the tomatoes in boiling water for a few seconds to loosen their skins, then peel, seed, and finely dice. Peel and finely chop the onions and peel and crush the garlic. Dry-fry the onions and garlic in a cooking pot, then add the thyme and the rosemary. Finely chop the bacon and add to the pot. Cook for a few minutes, then add the tomatoes. Add 2 tablespoons of water and cook over a low heat for 10 minutes. Set aside.

3 In a bowl, beat the egg and mix in the well-drained brocciu. Season with salt and pepper.

4 Remove the outer leaves from the artichokes, peel the stalks, and cut them off ½ in. (1 cm) from the heart. Cut off the top of the artichokes at two thirds of their height and rub them with the lemon. Spread the leaves out and put 1 tablespoon of brocciu in the center of each artichoke. Stand the artichokes up (stuffed side uppermost) in the cooking pot. Cover, and cook over a low heat for 1 hour until the artichokes are tender.

5 Break the crispbreads into a sealable plastic bag and crush using a rolling pin. To serve, sprinkle the crispbread topping over the artichokes and serve two to each person with some of the tomato and onion mixture.

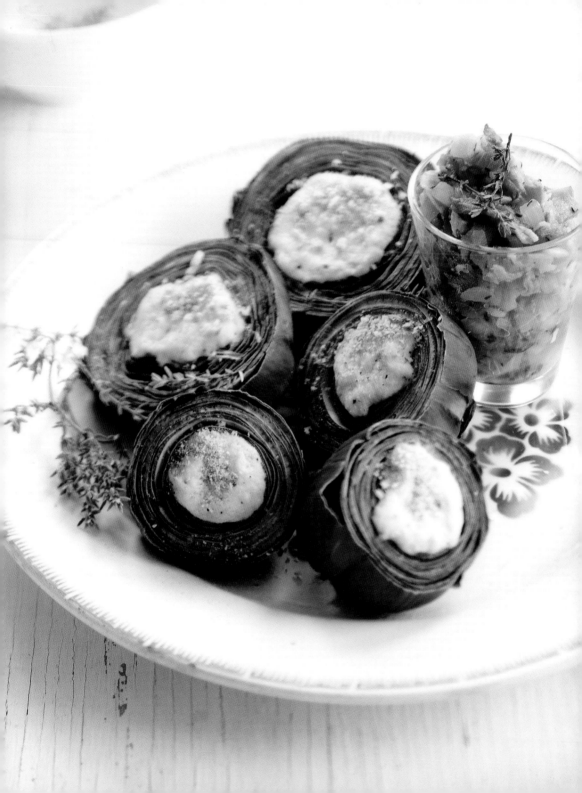

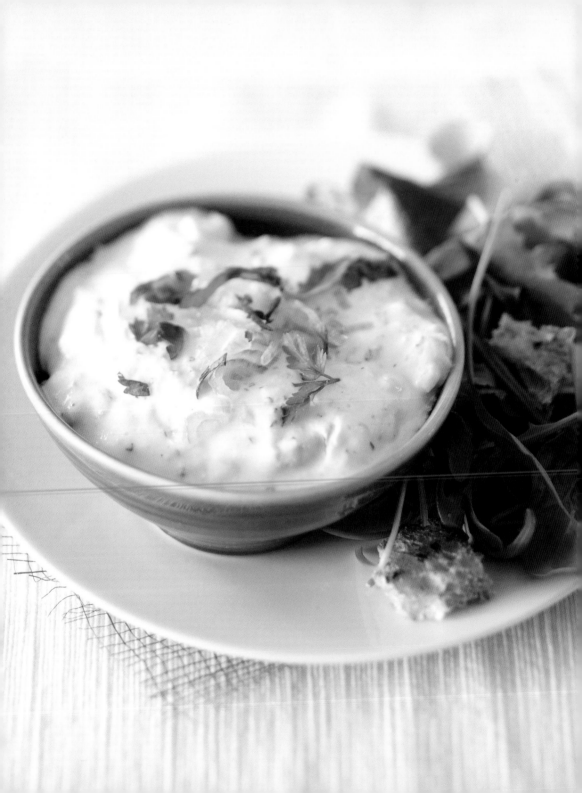

Lyonnaise cream cheese with herbs
Cervelle de canut

Don't be deceived: the French name for this dish—a specialty from Lyon—literally translated as "weavers' brains," makes reference to the silk-weavers of Lyon ("canuts"), who self-deprecatingly gave the name to this salad made from fresh fromage blanc. The calories in this recipe have been reduced by using nonfat fromage blanc (if unavailable, substitute plain nonfat yogurt), but it retains the same light texture by replacing salted whipped cream with whisked egg white.

PREP TIME 20 minutes | **CHILL TIME** 1 hour

INGREDIENTS FOR 4 PEOPLE
1 shallot
4 sprigs Italian (flat-leaf) parsley
4 sprigs chervil
1 ½ cups (14 oz./400 g) nonfat fromage blanc, or plain nonfat regular or Greek yogurt
2 tablespoons low-fat (3% fat) sour cream (crème fraîche)
1 teaspoon olive oil
1 teaspoon wine vinegar
1 tablespoon dry white wine
1 egg white
4 slices (2 oz./60 g) wholegrain bread
Salt and pepper

1 Peel and finely chop the shallot. Wash, dry, and chop the herbs.

2 Put the fromage blanc (or ricotta or cream cheese) in a salad bowl and whisk it. Add the cream and whisk together. Stir in the chopped shallot and herbs, then the oil, vinegar, wine, salt, and pepper. The mixture should be well seasoned.

3 In a separate bowl, whisk the egg white with a pinch of salt. Carefully fold it into the fromage blanc mixture. Refrigerate for 1 hour.

4 Toast the bread and cut it into cubes, then dry-fry the cubes to make croutons. Serve very cold on a bed of baby salad leaves with a few of the croutons.

Roast leg of lamb
Gigot d'agneau printanier

Traditionally eaten at Easter in France, leg of lamb is one of the best and leanest cuts of lamb. Roasted simply in the oven with various herbs and a fat-free stock, it retains all its tenderness without any extra fat.

PREP TIME 15 minutes | **COOK TIME** 30–45 minutes

INGREDIENTS FOR 4 PEOPLE
2 cloves garlic
1 ¼-lb. (600-g) leg of lamb, visible fat removed
4 teaspoons thyme leaves
4 teaspoons rosemary leaves
Zest of 2 untreated lemons
1 vegetable bouillon cube
1 teaspoon tomato paste (purée)
3 medium (14 oz./400g) tomatoes
Freshly ground pepper

1   Preheat the oven to 400°F (200°C/Gas mark 6).

2   Peel and slice the garlic cloves. Make cuts in the meat and poke slices of garlic into these slits. Place the joint in a roasting pan and sprinkle over the thyme, rosemary, and lemon zest. Place in the oven and roast for about 15 minutes.

3   Dissolve the bouillon cube in 1 cup (½ pint/250 ml) water and stir in the tomato paste. Cut the tomatoes in quarters. Remove the meat from the oven, pour the stock over, and arrange the tomato quarters around the meat. Grind over some pepper, then return the pan to the oven and cook for an additional 15–30 minutes, or until the lamb is cooked to your liking.

4   Serve hot.

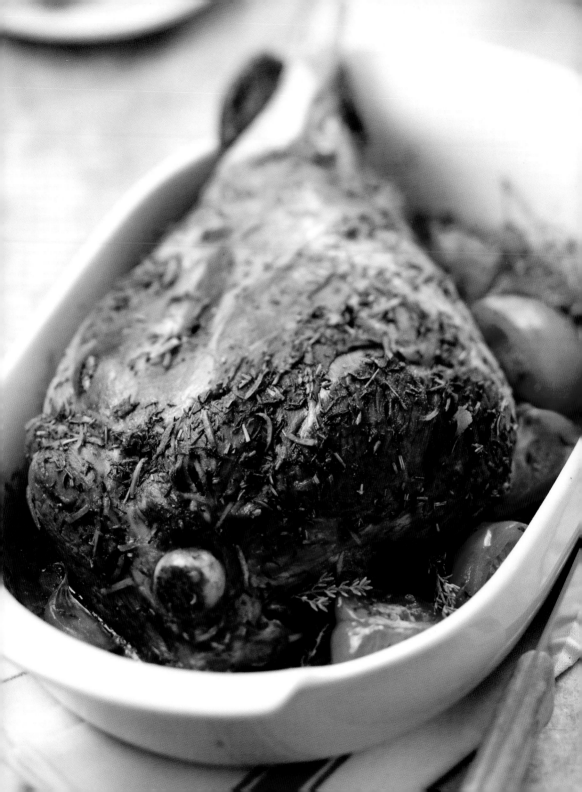

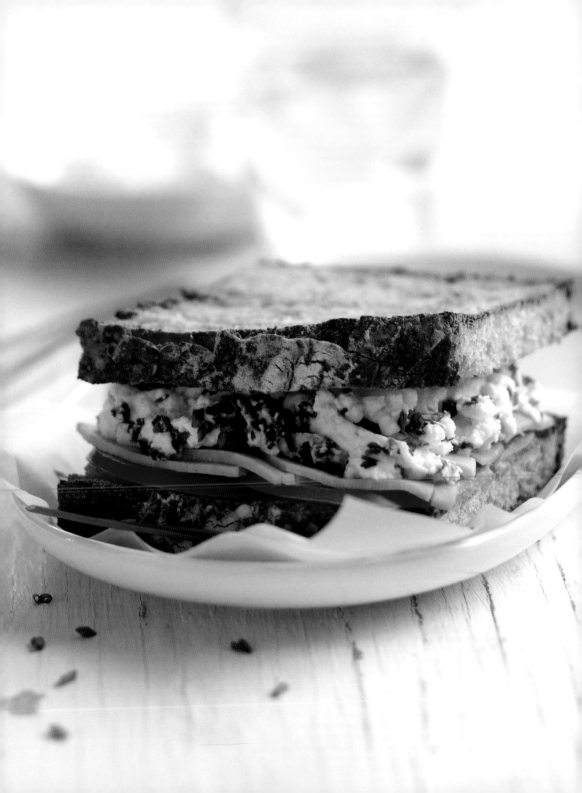

Croque-monsieur with fresh goat cheese
Croque-monsieur au chèvre frais

The favorite French toasted sandwich, the croque-monsieur is usually made from two slices of bread filled with ham, béchamel sauce (sometimes), and Swiss cheese, which is then broiled (grilled). To make a healthier version of this sandwich, use wholegrain or rye bread, which contain more fiber and less fat and sugar than commercial sliced bread. Adding tomato and using goat cheese rather than Swiss cheese reduces the fat content while retaining the calcium content.

PREP TIME 15 minutes | **COOK TIME** 5 minutes

INGREDIENTS FOR 4 PEOPLE
8 slices (¾ oz./20 g each) wholegrain or rye bread
4 teaspoons mustard
A few chives
5 ½ oz. (160 g) fresh goat cheese
2 slices lean ham
2 tomatoes
Freshly ground pepper

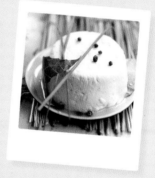

1   Toast the slices of bread. Spread each slice with mustard.

2   Wash and snip the chives. In a bowl mix together the fresh goat cheese, half the snipped chives, and some pepper, then spread it onto half the slices of toast.

3   Cut the ham into thin slices and divide it between these four toast slices. Wash and thinly slice the tomatoes and lay them on top of the ham.

4   Sprinkle over the remaining chopped chives and top with the remaining slices of toast. Serve on a bed of mixed salad leaves.

Stuffed tomatoes
Tomates à la farce légère

Every French family has its own favorite recipe for stuffed tomatoes, but as these recipes often contain sausage meat and bread crumbs, they're not always very healthy or light. By making the stuffing from a mixture of lean ground (minced) beef, lean ham, and prosciutto for a smoked taste, you'll reduce the amount of fat. Adding vegetables, such as mushrooms, to the stuffing also helps to reduce the calorific value of the dish.

PREP TIME 30 minutes | **COOK TIME** 45 minutes

INGREDIENTS FOR 4 PEOPLE

8 beefsteak tomatoes

3 ½ oz. (100 g) mushrooms

1 onion

2 cloves garlic

1 small bunch Italian (flat-leaf) parsley

2 slices lean ham

2 slices prosciutto, fat removed

14 oz. (400 g) lean ground (minced) beef (5% fat)

Pinch of *piment d'Espelette* (if unavailable, substitute cayenne pepper)

Salt and pepper

1 Preheat the oven to 400°F (200°C/Gas mark 6).

2 Wash the tomatoes, cut the top off each one, and scoop out the flesh. Reserve the "lids" and the flesh of two of the tomatoes. Salt the insides and place them upside down on a plate to drain.

3 Remove the end of the mushroom stalks and wipe the mushrooms with damp paper towels. Chop the mushrooms very finely, then dry-fry in a nonstick skillet (frying pan). Set aside. Peel the onion and garlic, wash the parsley, and blend in a food processor with the ham, prosciutto, and some of the reserved tomato (don't add too much as the stuffing needs to be sufficiently firm).

4 In a bowl, mix this stuffing mixture with the ground beef and the mushrooms. Season with salt, pepper, and *piment d'Espelette*. Fill the tomatoes with this mixture, place in a roasting pan, and bake in the oven for 40 minutes. Halfway through the cooking time, place the lids on the tomatoes in the pan.

5 Serve hot, two stuffed tomatoes per person.

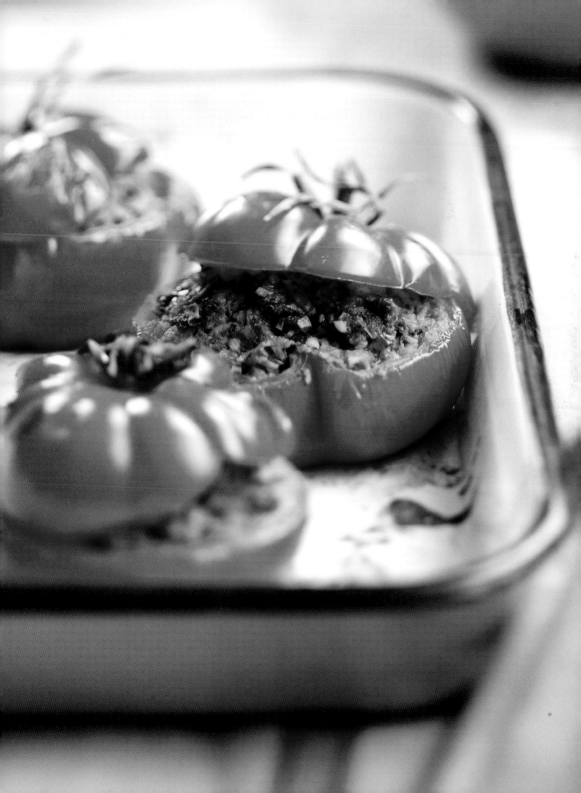

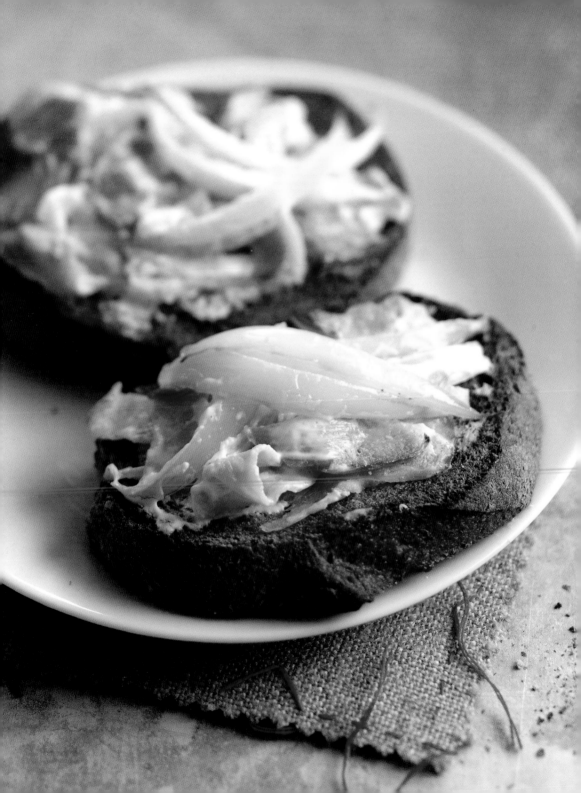

Alsatian open sandwiches
Tartines alsaciennes

Rediscover the tarte flambée, loved for being simple to make as well as for its taste. Replace the pastry with a thin slice of wholegrain toast, streaky bacon with lean smoked Canadian (back) bacon, and full-fat sour cream with nonfat fromage blanc or yogurt; you'll be able to enjoy this Alsatian specialty whenever you like as an appetizer or a main course, accompanied by a nice salad—in summer or winter.

PREP TIME 15 minutes | **COOK TIME** 15 minutes

INGREDIENTS FOR 4 PEOPLE

14 oz. (400 g) lean smoked Canadian-style (back) bacon
2 onions
8 thin slices (4 ¼ oz./120 g) wholegrain bread
Generous ¾ cup (7 oz./200 g) nonfat fromage
   blanc or plain nonfat regular or Greek yogurt
Salt and pepper

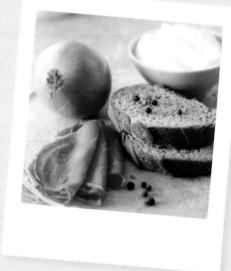

1 Cut the bacon into strips and dry-fry quickly in a nonstick skillet (frying pan), then set aside. Peel and slice the onions and sauté them in the same pan, adding a little water to deglaze the pan if necessary. Set aside.

2 Meanwhile, toast the bread slices.

3 Return the cooked bacon to the pan, remove from the heat, and stir in the fromage blanc or yogurt. Season with salt and pepper. Divide the bacon between the toast slices, top with the onion, and serve immediately.

Skate wings with capers
Ailes de raie à la grenobloise

This quick-and-easy recipe is a perfect way to discover and savor the fine flesh of skate. This light version of the classic Grenoble-style dish gives this fish a touch of acidity and sharpness without drowning it in butter.

PREP TIME 25 minutes | **COOK TIME** 20 minutes

INGREDIENTS FOR 4 PEOPLE
10 Italian (flat-leaf) parsley leaves
1 untreated lemon
4 slices (2 oz./60 g) wholegrain bread
4 pints (2 liters) fish stock
4 skate wings
1 tablespoon olive oil
¼ cup (1 ½ oz./40 g) capers
Salt and pepper

1 Wash and finely chop the parsley.

2 Remove the zest from the lemon using a vegetable peeler and set aside. Remove and discard all the pith and cut out the lemon segments.

3 Cut the bread into little cubes.

4 Heat the fish stock in a large cooking pot, add the skate wings and simmer for about 10 minutes until just cooked through.

5 Heat the olive oil in a nonstick skillet (frying pan) and fry the bread cubes, then add the capers and lemon zest and segments.

6 Place a skate wing on each plate and season with salt and pepper. Garnish with the crouton, caper, and lemon mixture, then sprinkle over the chopped parsley. Serve immediately.

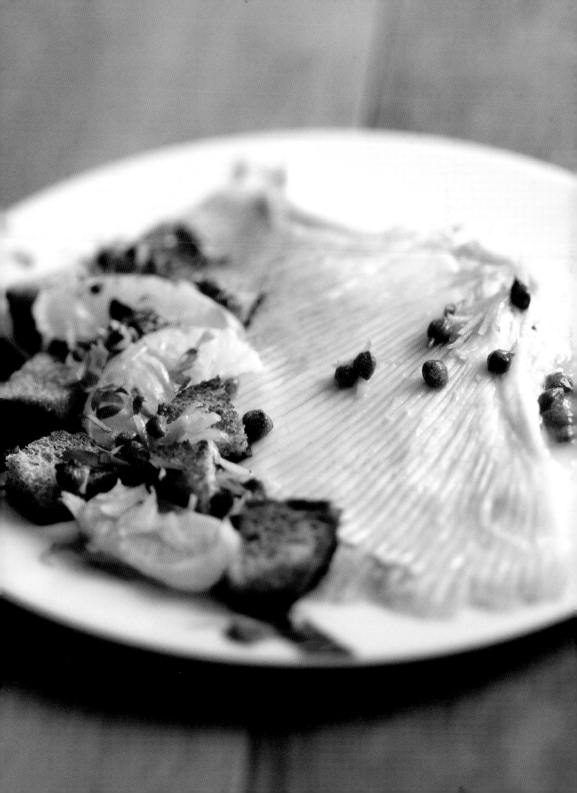

Veal blanquette
Blanquette de veau allégée

This classic of French cuisine is usually made with a white roux thinned down with stock and thickened with egg yolk and cream. This blanquette lightens the calorie load while retaining its subtle flavors. Choosing to use only cornstarch (cornflour) and low-fat sour cream (crème fraîche) will mean that you can confidently enjoy this fine dish.

PREP TIME 35 minutes | **COOK TIME** 2 hours

INGREDIENTS FOR 4 PEOPLE

1 ¼ lb. (600 g) lean stewing veal

2 onions

2 cloves garlic

1 carrot

1 veal bouillon cube (if unavailable, substitute a chicken bouillon cube)

1 sprig thyme

1 bay leaf

1 lb. (500 g) mushrooms

2 tablespoons cornstarch (cornflour)

1 teaspoon mustard

4 tablespoons low-fat sour cream (crème fraîche)

Salt and pepper

1 Cube the meat and brown it in a nonstick skillet (frying pan) without adding fat. Peel and finely chop the onions. Add them to the pan and continue to cook over a low heat.

2 Peel and finely chop the garlic, add it and cook for an additional few minutes over a low heat. Peel and thickly slice the carrot and add it to the pan. Season with salt and pepper and cover with water. Add the bouillon cube, thyme, and bay leaf, cover, and simmer for 1 ½ hours.

3 Wipe the mushrooms with damp paper towels, remove the end of the stalks, then chop the mushrooms, add to the pan, and cook for an additional 15 minutes. Strain, reserving the cooking liquid.

4 Off the heat, pour the cooking liquid gradually over the cornstarch, stirring constantly to prevent lumps forming. Pour the sauce back into the pan over a low heat and stir constantly until it thickens. Stir in the mustard and sour cream. Return the meat and vegetables to the pan and heat for an additional 5 minutes over a low heat.

5 Serve hot.

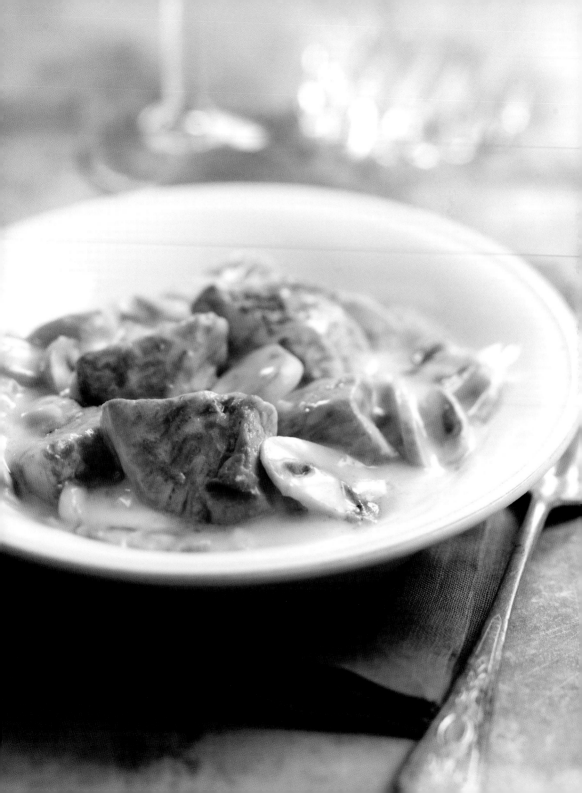

Navarin of lamb
Navarin d'agneau minceur

Navarin is, according to the etymology of the word, a dish based around turnips. More precisely, it is a lamb and vegetable stew. Because lamb is a fatty meat, it is important to choose the piece carefully and to avoid using fat when cooking.

PREP TIME 35 minutes | **COOK TIME** 1 hour 40 minutes

INGREDIENTS FOR 4 PEOPLE
1 ¾ lb. (800 g) lean lamb, visible fat removed
2 cloves garlic
2 cups (1 pint/500 ml) veal stock
3 tablespoons all-purpose (plain) flour
14-oz. (400-g) can crushed (chopped) tomatoes
1 bay leaf
1 teaspoon thyme leaves
14 oz. (400 g) carrots
9 oz. (250 g) turnips
8 baby onions
Salt and pepper

1 Chop the lamb into 2-in. (5-cm) cubes. Brown the meat in a nonstick cooking pot over a medium heat without adding fat, to obtain the juices.

2 Peel and crush the garlic cloves, add them to the pot, and continue cooking.

3 Heat the stock. Toss the diced lamb in the flour seasoned with salt and pepper, making sure it is thoroughly coated. Cook for a few minutes until the flour has turned golden brown. Pour the stock over the meat while stirring. Add the tomatoes, bay leaf, and thyme. Simmer, covered, for 50 minutes over a medium heat.

4 Wash and peel the carrots and turnips. Cut the turnips into large cubes and thickly slice the carrots. Peel the baby onions. Add the turnips, carrots, and onions to the pot, reduce the heat, and continue cooking for an additional 30 minutes.

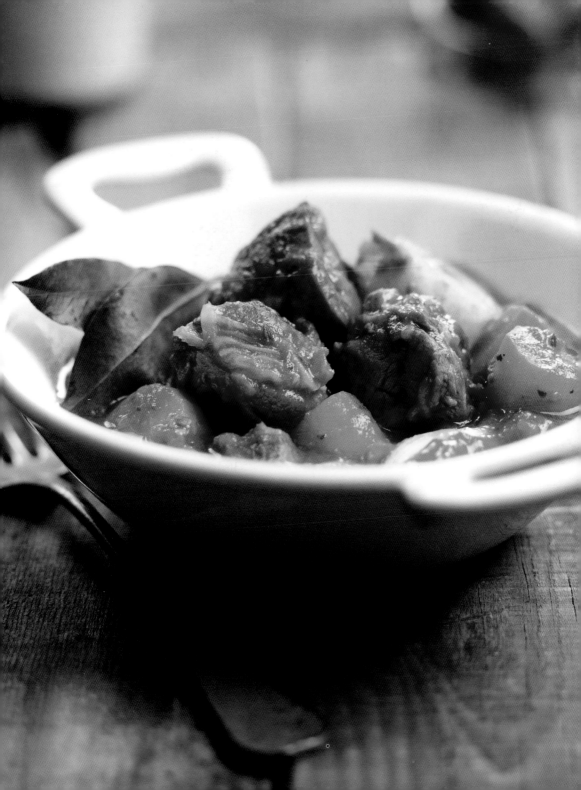

Bordeaux-style porcini
Cèpes à la bordelaise

A delicious mushroom with a sweet nutty flavor, the porcini is a staple of French cuisine. But you need to know how to prepare it, other than the traditional method of frying it in lots of oil. Here, a teaspoon of oil is all that's needed: the aromatics do the rest!

PREP TIME 20 minutes | **COOK TIME** 15 minutes

INGREDIENTS FOR 4 PEOPLE
1 lb. (500 g) porcini
2 small shallots
2 cloves garlic
2 tablespoons chopped parsley
3 crispbreads or 3 slices of stale bread
1 teaspoon olive oil
2 tablespoons lemon juice
Salt and pepper

1 Separate the caps from the stalks of the porcini. Remove and discard the ends of the stalks, then carefully wipe the caps and stalks using damp paper towels. Peel the shallots and garlic.

2 Finely mince the porcini stalks, shallots, parsley, garlic, and crispbreads or stale bread.

3 Heat the teaspoon of oil in a skillet (frying pan) and cook the porcini caps over a very low heat, being careful not to let them brown. When they're half cooked, move them to the edges of the pan and add the minced mushroom mixture to the center. Cook gently for 5 minutes, stirring occasionally. Season with salt and pepper and sprinkle with lemon juice.

4 Lay the mushroom caps on a plate and cover them with the minced mushrooms. Serve.

Rabbit with mustard
Lapin à la moutarde

Rabbit is an often-forgotten meat, yet it is particularly lean, fine, and much less expensive than red meat or veal. Cooking it in a well-flavored sauce—here with mustard—retains all its tenderness and gives it character.

PREP TIME 20 minutes | **COOK TIME** 45 minutes

INGREDIENTS FOR 4 PEOPLE
8 saddles of rabbit (1 ¼ lb./600 g total)
4 tablespoons traditional wholegrain mustard
2 shallots
8 large tomatoes
Salt and pepper

1 Trim the saddles of rabbit if necessary, cut into pieces, and brush them generously with mustard.

2 Peel and finely chop the shallots. Peel and slice the tomatoes. Dry-fry the shallots in a nonstick skillet (frying pan) until transparent, then add the sliced tomatoes. Season with salt and pepper and add the saddles of rabbit. Cook for about 35 minutes, covered, stirring occasionally.

3 Serve hot.

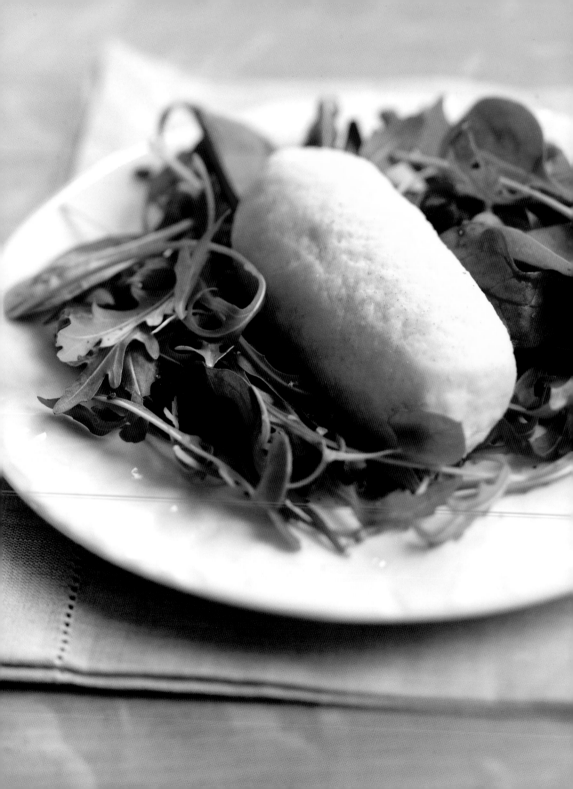

Pike quenelles
Quenelles de brochet légères

This Lyonnaise specialty usually includes flour or durum wheat semolina. Without carbohy-drates, this recipe is lighter. Pike reveals its true taste and you benefit from its low-fat and high-protein content.

PREP TIME 40 minutes | **COOK TIME** 15 minutes

INGREDIENTS FOR 4 PEOPLE
14 oz. (400 g) raw pike meat
1 whole egg + 1 egg white
Scant ½ cup (3 ½ fl. oz./100 ml) light half-and-half (single cream)
Pinch of grated nutmeg
Salt and white pepper

1 Carefully remove any small bones and pieces of skin that you might find in the pike meat.

2 In a bowl, whisk the egg white to peak stage with a pinch of salt. Set aside.

3 Place the pike meat, whole egg, cream, nutmeg, and salt and pepper in a food processor and chop finely. Fold in the whisked egg white using a spatula. Divide the mixture into four equal portions.

4 Spread out some heatproof plastic wrap on the work surface. Place a portion of the mixture at one end of the plastic wrap and begin to roll it to form a sausage. Hold the end of the sausage with one hand and with the other hand flat, roll the sausage forward to tighten the stuffing in the sausage. Make a knot at either end to seal the sausage. Repeat with the other three portions of mixture.

5 Fill a large saucepan with water and bring to a boil. When it is boiling, drop the four pike packages into the water. Cook for 15 minutes.

6 Drain the packages and cut the knot from one end of each. Slide the quenelles out onto a clean dish cloth (tea towel) to mop up any excess liquid.

7 Serve one pike quenelle per person, accompanied, if desired, by 1 tablespoon of a reduced shellfish broth and a small mixed baby leaf salad.

French toast with fresh fruit
Pain perdu aux fruits

French toast is a simple and cheap dish to prepare, so why deprive yourself? Made with fat-free milk and cooked without fat, it will easily fit in your diet. Add slices of fresh fruit and a note of cinnamon for a truly delicious dessert.

PREP TIME 10 minutes | **COOK TIME** 10 minutes | **CHILL TIME** 5 minutes

INGREDIENTS FOR 4 PEOPLE
2 eggs
1 cup (½ pint/240 ml) fat-free milk
2 teaspoons honey
1 teaspoon ground cinnamon
Fresh fruit of your choice
Juice of ½ lemon
4 oz. (115 g) stale or slightly toasted bread
1 teaspoon peanut (groundnut) oil

1   Whisk the eggs in a bowl and pour them into a shallow dish.

2   In another shallow dish, mix together the milk, honey, and cinnamon.

3   Peel (if necessary) and chop the fruit. Sprinkle with lemon juice, cover with plastic wrap, and refrigerate.

4   Cut the bread into eight thin slices. Heat the oil in a nonstick skillet (frying pan). Quickly dip the bread slices, one at a time, in the milk, then in the egg, making sure both sides are coated. Fry them in the pan until golden brown on both sides.

5   Remove them to individual plates and top with the prepared fruit. Serve immediately.

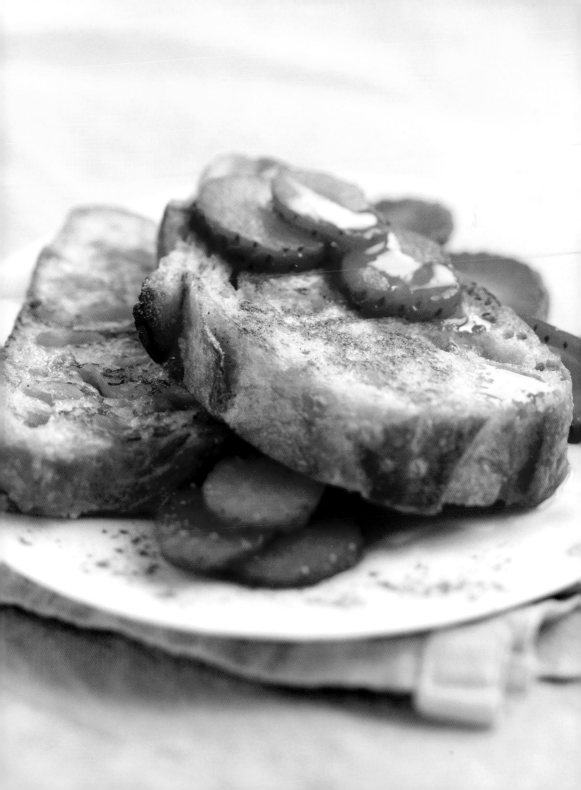

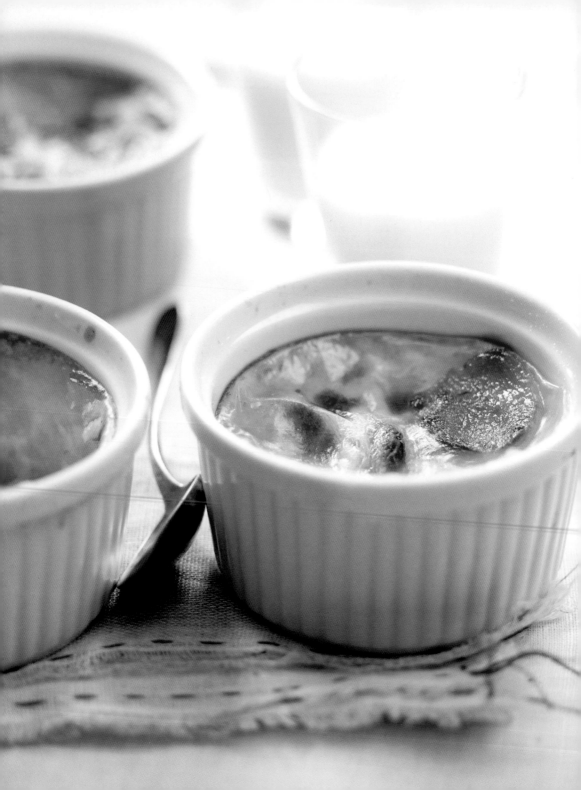

Apricot custards
Flans aux abricots

There are many variations of custard as a dessert, including caramel custard and custard tart. This one contains dried apricots, which are available year round, but you could also use fresh fruits, depending on your taste and what's in season.

PREP TIME 15 minutes | **CHILL TIME** 15 minutes | **COOK TIME** 45 minutes

INGREDIENTS FOR 4 PEOPLE
½ cup (3 oz./80 g) dried apricots
1 ⅔ cups (13 ½ fl. oz./400 ml) fat-free milk
½ vanilla bean (pod)
2 eggs
2 tablespoons powdered sweetener for cooking
¼ cup (1 ½ oz./40 g) cornstarch (cornflour)

1   Preheat the oven to 350°F (180°C/Gas mark 4).

2   Rehydrate the apricots in the microwave with a little water, cut them in half, then divide them between four ramekins and refrigerate.

3   Put the milk and the split and scraped vanilla bean into a saucepan and bring to a boil.

4   In a bowl, whisk the eggs with the sweetener until the mixture pales. Sift in the cornstarch and stir to mix in. Remove the vanilla bean from the milk. Pour the milk over the eggs, stirring vigorously. Pour the mixture back into the pan and heat over a low heat for 2 minutes, stirring constantly.

5   Pour this cream over the chilled apricots and bake in the oven for 30 minutes.

6   Serve warm or cold.

Pineapple soufflé
Soufflé à l'ananas

A soufflé is guaranteed to impress your guests when you serve it up. To enjoy it guilt-free, make this sweet version, which includes pineapple for an exotic touch and won't show up on your waistline because it's made with fat-free milk.

PREP TIME 30 minutes | **COOK TIME** 45 minutes

INGREDIENTS FOR 4 PEOPLE
Scant 1 cup (7 fl. oz./200 ml) fat-free milk
2 eggs
2 tablespoons powdered sweetener for cooking
2 tablespoons (¾ oz./20 g) cornstarch (cornflour)
½ pineapple

1 Preheat the oven to 350°F (180°C/Gas mark 4). Line a soufflé dish with parchment (greaseproof) paper.

2 Heat the milk in a saucepan. Separate the egg whites and yolks into two bowls and set aside the whites. Whisk the egg yolks with 1 tablespoon of sweetener until the mixture becomes thicker, pale, and leaves a trail. Sift in the cornstarch and stir to mix in. Pour the hot milk gradually over the egg yolks, stirring. Pour the mixture back into the pan and bring to a boil, stirring constantly, then transfer it to a mixing bowl.

3 Peel the pineapple, remove its hard core, and blend to a purée in a food processor. Stir the pineapple purée into the egg yolk mixture.

4 Whisk the egg whites until they form peaks, adding the remaining 1 tablespoon of sweetener to "stabilize" the whites. Gently fold them into the pineapple cream. Pour this mixture into the soufflé dish until two thirds full, then bake in the oven for 25 minutes.

5 Serve immediately.

Floating islands with mint crème anglaise
Îles flottantes, crème à la menthe

Îles flottantes are a classic French dessert, composed of poached egg whites "floating" in a light custard sauce (crème anglaise). This variation, made with fat-free milk and sweetener, can be enjoyed with a clear conscience and will surprise your guests with its original mint-flavored crème anglaise.

PREP TIME 30 minutes | **COOK TIME** 15 minutes | **CHILL TIME** 25 minutes

INGREDIENTS FOR 4 PEOPLE
½ bunch mint
1 ⅔ cups (13 ½ fl. oz./400 ml) fat-free milk
3 whole eggs + 1 egg white
4 tablespoons powdered sweetener for cooking
Pinch of salt

1　Wash the mint leaves. Reserve a few leaves for decoration and finely chop the remainder. Put the milk into a saucepan with the chopped mint and bring to a boil. Remove from the heat and set aside to infuse.

2　Separate the egg whites and yolks into two bowls. Set aside the whites. Whisk the egg yolks with 2 tablespoons of sweetener until the mixture becomes pale. Strain the milk and add to the whisked egg yolks, stirring constantly. Pour the mixture back into the pan and heat over a very low heat, stirring constantly using a wooden spoon. The crème anglaise is ready when it coats the back of the spoon. Refrigerate until ready to serve.

3　Using an electric whisk, whisk the egg whites with a pinch of salt until they form stiff peaks. Add the remaining 2 tablespoons of sweetener to "stabilize" the whites (so that they retain their volume).

4　Bring a little water to a boil in a large saucepan, then reduce the heat so that the water is at a gentle simmer. Shape eight small quenelles from the egg whites using two tablespoons. Gently lower the quenelles into the water and poach them for about 1 minute on each side.

5　Divide the mint crème anglaise between four small dessert bowls, arrange two quenelles in each, and decorate with a few mint leaves.

Vanilla ice cream
Glace légère à la vanille

Vanilla ice cream is made with cream, milk, egg yolks, and sugar. It's impossible to imagine a summer without ice creams and sundaes, so to take advantage of this unmissable, refreshing dessert during the summertime, make this ice cream yourself from a light vanilla custard.

PREP TIME 15 minutes | **COOK TIME** 15 minutes | **FREEZE TIME** 3 hours

INGREDIENTS FOR 4 PEOPLE
2 cups (1 pint/500 ml) fat-free milk
1 vanilla bean (pod)
3 egg yolks
1 teaspoon cornstarch (cornflour)
4 teaspoons powdered sweetener for cooking
2 tablespoons low-fat (3% fat) sour cream (crème fraîche)

1   Put the milk in a saucepan with the split and scraped vanilla bean and place over a gentle heat.

2   In a large bowl, whisk the egg yolks with the cornstarch using an electric whisk until they thicken and turn pale.

3   Strain the milk and slowly pour it over the whisked egg yolks, stirring constantly. Heat over a gentle heat, stirring constantly, until it begins to thicken slightly (it should have the texture of crème anglaise). Stir in the sweetener and the cream.

4   Pour into a freezer-proof container. Place in the freezer and stir every 20 minutes with a fork, until the ice cream is frozen. Alternatively, use an ice-cream maker.

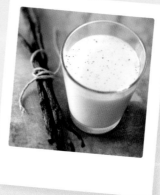

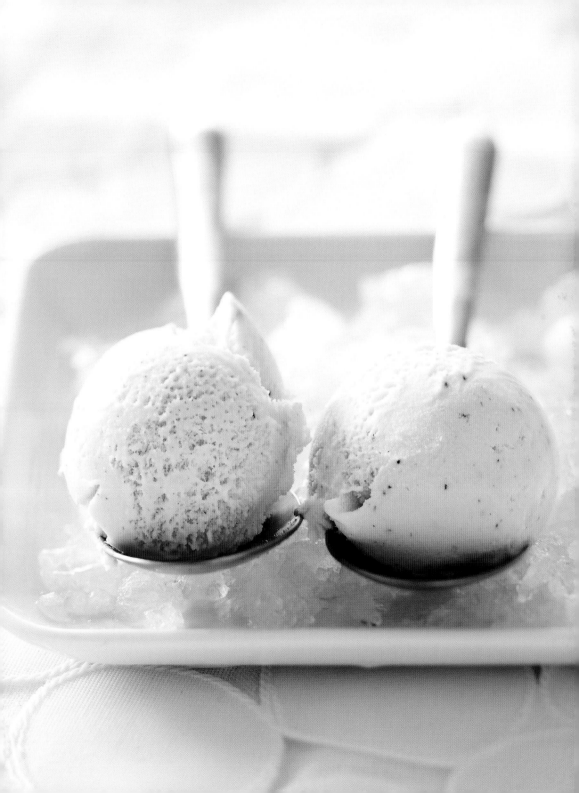

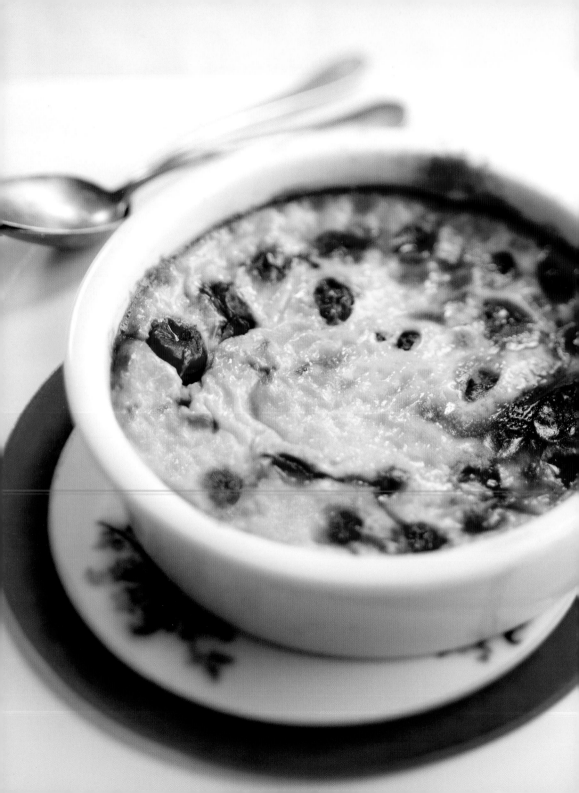

Morello-cherry clafoutis
Clafoutis léger aux griottes

Clafoutis is a dessert originating from the Limousin region of France. Traditionally it contains unpitted cherries, but you can eat it any time of year in the form of "flognarde," varying the fruits—try apple or pear—according to what's in season. Made without butter, this recipe can easily be incorporated into your diet.

PREP TIME 15 minutes | **COOK TIME** 20 minutes

INGREDIENTS FOR 4 PEOPLE
1 ⅔ cups (13 ½ fl. oz./400 ml) fat-free milk
3 eggs
4 teaspoons powdered sweetener for cooking
¼ cup (1 ½ oz./40 g) cornstarch (cornflour)
14 oz. (400 g) morello cherries, fresh, or canned and drained

1 Preheat the oven to 400°F (200°C/Gas mark 6).

2 Lightly warm the milk.

3 Using an electric whisk, beat the eggs with the sweetener in a bowl, then sift in the cornstarch and stir until you have a smooth batter. Gradually add the milk, stirring well to avoid the mixture forming lumps.

4 Line a springform pan (cake tin) with parchment (greaseproof) paper, pour in the batter and sprinkle the cherries over the top. Bake in the oven for 20 minutes.

Apricot charlotte
Charlotte aux abricots

Even in its original version, the charlotte is a fairly light dessert because it is rich in fruits and low in fat. But we've reduced the calories even further by using low-fat sour cream.

PREP TIME 40 minutes | **FREEZE TIME** 15 minutes | **CHILL TIME** 8 hours

INGREDIENTS FOR 4 PEOPLE
Scant 1 cup (7 fl. oz./200 ml) low-fat sour cream (crème fraîche)
1 lb. 5 oz. (600 g) canned apricots in syrup
1 tablespoon rum
18 ladyfingers (sponge fingers)
1 leaf (¹⁄₁₆ oz./2 g) gelatin
1 tablespoon crushed ice
Pinch of salt
2 sticks (⅛ oz./4 g) vanilla sweetener

1 Place the sour cream in the freezer for 15 minutes.

2 Drain the apricots, reserving the syrup. In a shallow dish, mix this syrup with the rum. Soak the ladyfingers in the syrup, then arrange them in the base and around the sides of a charlotte mold.

3 Soak the gelatin in a small bowl of cold water, then remove it, squeeze it out, and dissolve it in 2 tablespoons of warm water. Let cool.

4 Beat the cold sour cream with the crushed ice, salt, and vanilla sweetener. Stir in the gelatin.

5 Chop the apricots into small pieces. Fill the charlotte mold with alternating layers of whipped cream and chopped apricots. Set aside any remaining whipped cream and apricots in the refrigerator to use as decoration. Place the charlotte in the refrigerator overnight.

6 To serve, unmold onto a plate and decorate with any remaining whipped cream and apricots.

Vacherin

This frozen dessert is easy to digest at the end of a festive meal. We have chosen to lighten the ice cream but it remains a delicious, refreshing, and fruity recipe.

PREP TIME 45 minutes | **FREEZE TIME** 10 hours

INGREDIENTS FOR 4 PEOPLE
⅔ cup (5 fl. oz./150 ml) half-and-half (single cream)
2 eggs
2 teaspoons powdered sweetener
2 tablespoons superfine (caster) sugar
1 stick (¹⁄₁₆ oz./2 g) vanilla sweetener
1 teaspoon vanilla extract
Scant ½ cup (3 ½ fl. oz./100 ml) raspberry coulis (if unavailable,
    make your own using 1 ½ cups (8 oz./225 g) raspberries + 2 tablespoons water)
2 large meringues

1 Pour the cream into a bowl and freeze for 30 minutes.

2 Separate the egg whites from the yolks. In a mixing bowl, whisk the egg yolks, the unfla-
   vored sweetener, and the sugar.

3 Remove the cream from the freezer, add the vanilla sweetener, and whip. When the cream
   is well whipped (at least 5 minutes), add the vanilla extract, while continuing to whisk.

4 In another bowl, whisk the egg whites until they form peaks. Lifting the mixture with
   a spoon, carefully fold the whisked egg whites into the yolks, then fold in the whipped
   cream. Don't overmix or the mousse will collapse.

5 If making your own coulis, place the raspberries in a food processor or blender with the
   water and liquidize until a very smooth coulis is obtained. Strain through a chinois (fine
   sieve) to remove any seeds. If necessary, add a little sweetener to taste. Pour the raspberry
   coulis into a cake pan, then coarsely crumble the meringues over the top to half fill the
   mold. Finally, spoon over the cream mixture. Freeze overnight.

6 Turn the *vacherin* out of the mold onto a plate and serve.

Peach Melba verrines
Pêches en verrines façon Melba

Traditionally, peach Melba is comprised of peaches poached in syrup accompanied by vanilla ice cream, raspberry sauce, and often sweetened whipped cream. There are several variations: strawberry Melba, for example. This variation on the classic, which is served in a glass and marries peaches with iced vanilla-flavored nonfat fromage blanc (if unavailable, use plain nonfat yogurt), will satisfy those with a sweet tooth without proving a heavy finish to a meal.

PREP TIME 20 minutes | **CHILL TIME** 15 minutes | **FREEZE TIME** 8 hours

INGREDIENTS FOR 4 PEOPLE
½ vanilla bean (pod)
1 cup (8 ½ oz./240 g) nonfat fromage blanc, or plain nonfat regular or Greek yogurt
2 teaspoons powdered sweetener
8 canned peach halves, drained
4 teaspoons raspberry Jell-O or gelatin dessert
2 tablespoons sliced (flaked) almonds, toasted (optional)

1 Split the vanilla bean in half lengthwise and scrape the seeds into a bowl. Stir in the fromage blanc (or yogurt) and the powdered sweetener and set aside in the refrigerator.

2 Dice the peach halves and set aside in the refrigerator.

3 Put the raspberry Jell-O into a ramekin, add 3 tablespoons of water, heat in the microwave for 1 minute, then stir until smooth.

4 Put some diced peach in each of four straight-sided clear glasses, top with some vanilla-flavored fromage blanc, spoon over some raspberry Jell-O, then repeat these layers. Place the verrines in the freezer for 30 minutes.

5 If desired, decorate with toasted sliced almonds (dry-fried in a pan). Serve immediately.

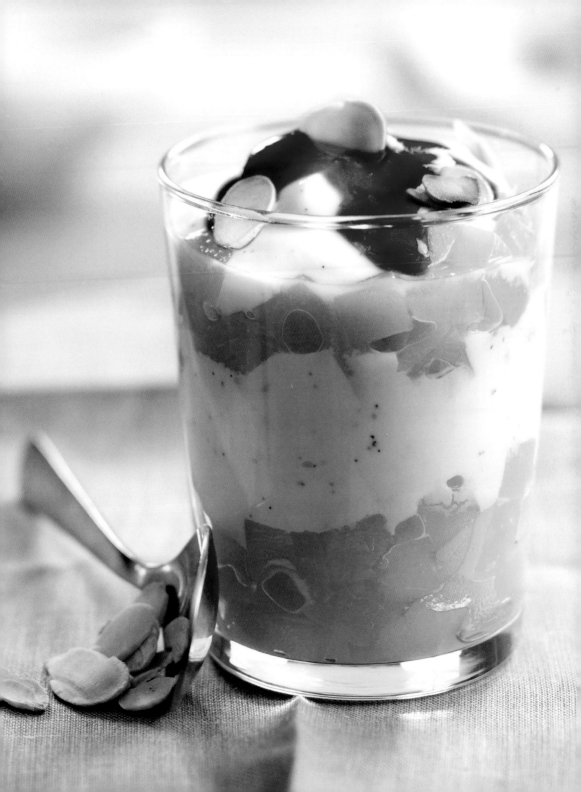

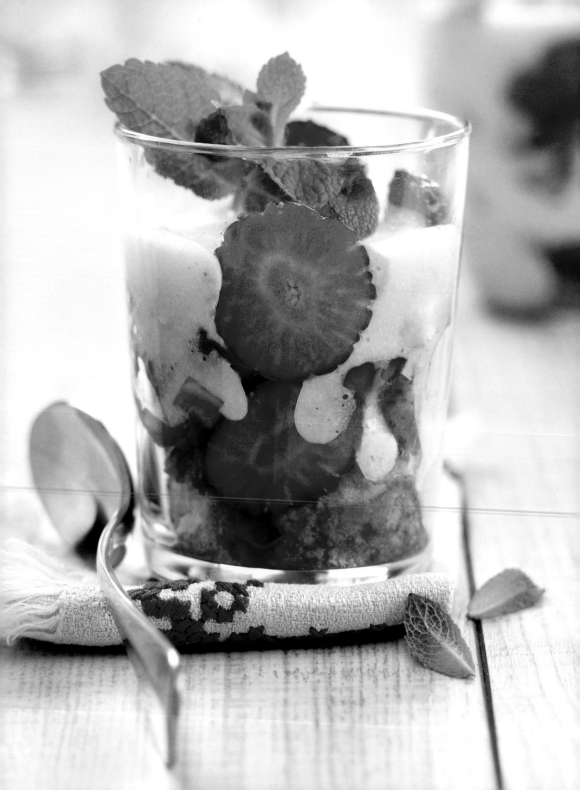

Strawberry verrines
Verrines façon fraisier

A fraisier is a gâteau made with sponge cake and crème mousseline *(a mixture of* crème patissière *and butter). To enjoy this classic guilt-free, try this verrine—a delight to look at as well as to taste—which combines a light, butter-free whipped cream made with a reasonable quantity of ladyfingers (sponge fingers) and lots of strawberries!*

PREP TIME 40 minutes | **COOK TIME** 10 minutes | **CHILL TIME** 1 hour

INGREDIENTS FOR 4 PEOPLE

Scant 1 cup (7 fl. oz./200 ml) fat-free milk
½ vanilla bean (pod)
1 egg
2 tablespoons powdered sweetener for cooking
1 ½ tablespoons (½ oz./15 g) cornstarch (cornflour)
1 teaspoon kirsch
Pinch of salt

9 oz. (250 g) fresh strawberries
1 teaspoon strawberry coulis (if
    unavailable, make your own using
    1 ½ cups/8 oz./225 g fresh strawberries
    + 1 tbs lemon juice + 1 tbs water)
12 ladyfingers (sponge fingers)
A few fresh mint leaves

1   Put the milk and the split and scraped vanilla bean into a saucepan and bring to a boil. Remove from the heat and set aside to infuse.

2   Separate the egg white and yolk and set aside the white. In a bowl, whisk the egg yolk with the sweetener until the mixture pales. Sift in the cornstarch and stir to mix in. Slowly strain the hot milk over the whisked egg yolk, stirring constantly. Pour back into the pan and heat gently, stirring, until the mixture begins to thicken. Remove from the heat and stir in the kirsch. Using an electric whisk, whisk the egg white with a pinch of salt until it forms stiff peaks. Gently fold it into the cream.

3   Wash and hull the strawberries. Cut 20 of them in half and finely dice the remainder. If making your own coulis, place the strawberries in a food processor or blender with the lemon juice and water and liquidize until a very smooth coulis is obtained. Strain through a chinois (fine sieve) to remove any seeds. If necessary, add a little sweetener to taste. In a shallow dish, mix the strawberry coulis with 3 tablespoons of water. Dip the ladyfingers in this syrup, then cut them in half crosswise. Place three ladyfinger halves in the bottom of four straight-sided clear glasses, arrange five strawberry halves around the edge of the glass, spoon in some *crème mousseline*, then top with some of the diced strawberries. Repeat these layers. Refrigerate for 1 hour.

4   Decorate with some chopped mint leaves before serving.

Avocado and shrimp salad
Rosaces d'avocat cœur de crevettes

Avocado is a fruit that is high in fat (22 percent), but you can still include it in a weight-loss diet as long as you avoid calorific mayonnaise and opt instead for a light dressing that will compensate for its richness. Try this revisited, light version of avocados with shrimp (prawns)—a dish you might have thought was banned forever.

PREP TIME 15 minutes | **CHILL TIME** 15 minutes

INGREDIENTS FOR 4 PEOPLE

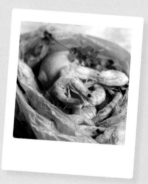

14 oz. (400 g) peeled and cooked fresh
   shrimp (prawns)
1 small bunch cilantro (coriander)
1 shallot
2 plain nonfat petits-suisses, or 4 tablespoons
   (2 oz./55 g) fat-free cottage cheese + 3 tablespoons
   (1 ½ oz./45 g) plain nonfat Greek yogurt
Juice of 1 lemon
2 very ripe avocados
Salt and pepper

1 Cut the shrimp into small pieces. Finely chop the fresh cilantro, reserving a few leaves for decoration. Peel and finely chop the shallot. Drain the petits-suisses (or cottage cheese) well. Put in a bowl with the shrimp, cilantro, petits-suisses (or cottage cheese and Greek yogurt), and the juice of half the lemon, and stir to combine. Season with salt and pepper. Divide the mixture between four individual ramekins and refrigerate until required.

2 Peel the avocados, cut them in half, and remove the pit. Finely slice each avocado half and arrange it in a fan shape around the edge of four small plates, like the petals of a flower. Sprinkle with the remaining lemon juice.

3 Remove the ramekins from the refrigerator and turn them out onto the center of each plate.

4 Decorate each plate with a few of the reserved cilantro leaves and serve chilled.

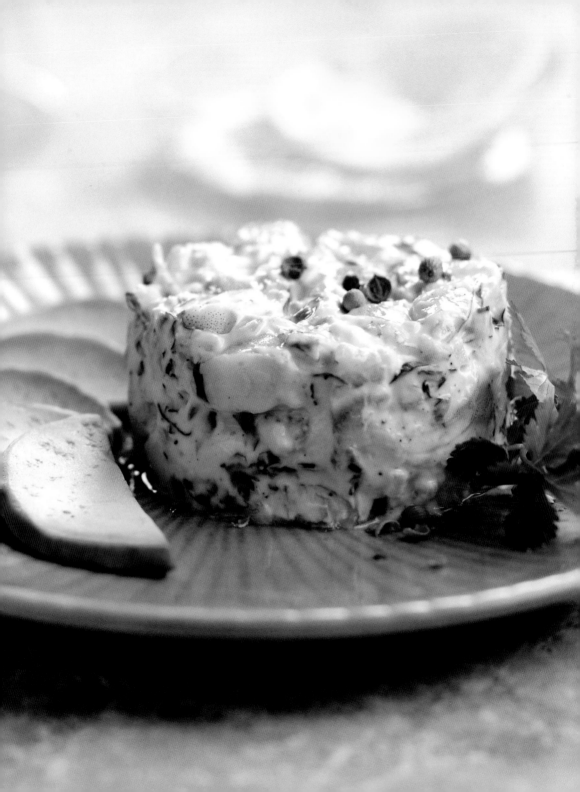

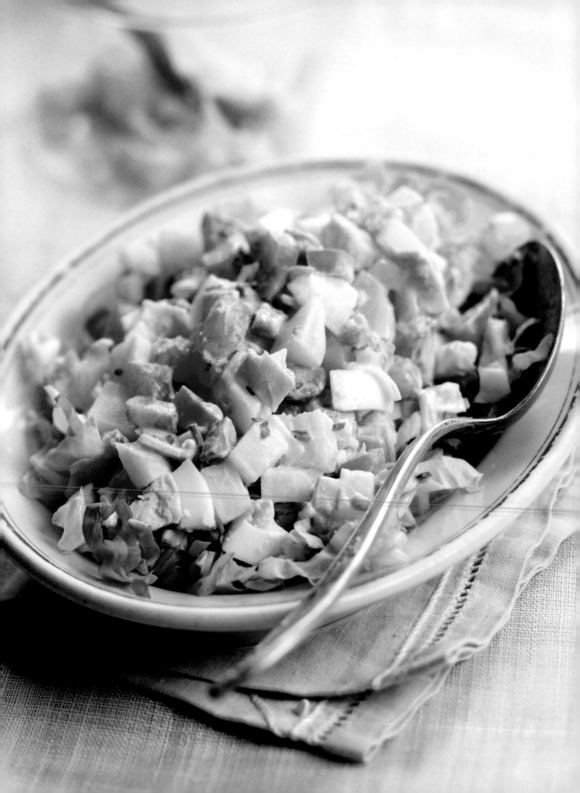

Potato and ham salad
Salade fraîche à la piémontaise

With potatoes, ham, hard-boiled eggs, and mayonnaise, this famous French salad often loses out when you're trying to watch your weight. But this homemade recipe—which combines just the right proportions with a fresh dressing made from nonfat fromage blanc (if unavailable, substitute plain nonfat yogurt)—will enable you to enjoy this traditional salad at buffets and picnics with a clear conscience.

PREP TIME 25 minutes | **COOK TIME** 15 minutes | **CHILL TIME** 25 minutes

INGREDIENTS FOR 4 PEOPLE
14 oz. (400 g) waxy potatoes (e.g. Charlotte)
2 eggs
2 small white onions
8 fresh chives
Scant 1 cup (7 oz./200 g) nonfat fromage blanc or plain nonfat
    regular or Greek yogurt
1 heaped teaspoon mustard
1 tablespoon lemon juice
14 oz. (400 g) tomatoes
8 small pickles (pickled gherkins)
7 oz. (200 g) lean ham
7 oz. (200 g) lettuce
Salt and pepper

1   An hour ahead, wash, peel, and steam the potatoes until tender when pierced with the tip of a sharp knife. Hard-boil the eggs and let cool.

2   Prepare the dressing. Peel and finely chop the onions. Rinse and snip the chives. In a bowl, mix together the fromage blanc or yogurt, mustard, lemon juice, chives, and onion. Season with salt and pepper and refrigerate.

3   Dice the potatoes, tomatoes, hard-boiled eggs, and pickles, and mix together in a bowl. Cut the ham into thin strips and stir into the salad along with the fromage blanc or cream cheese dressing. Mix well.

4   Wash and trim the salad leaves and divide between four small plates. Spoon the salad over the bed of lettuce on each plate and serve chilled.

73

Rillettes

Ah, charcuterie! You love it but you know you need to limit yourself to small portions and it's difficult to stick to them. That's why we've included this recipe for rillettes, which has the merit of being made with lean meat.

PREP TIME 20 minutes | **COOK TIME** 15 minutes | **CHILL TIME** 1 hour

INGREDIENTS FOR 4 PEOPLE
9 oz. (250 g) pork tenderloin (fillet)
Scant ½ cup (3 ½ oz./100 g) low-fat sour cream (crème fraîche)
1 teaspoon Tabasco
1 teaspoon mild mustard
1 clove garlic
A few snipped chives
Salt and pepper

1 Dice the pork tenderloin and sauté it in a nonstick skillet (frying pan) without adding fat. Let cool.

2 Blend well in a food processor with the cream, Tabasco, mustard, garlic, salt, and pepper until the mixture is smooth. Stir in the snipped chives.

3 Pour the mixture into a small terrine dish and smooth the surface with a spatula. Set aside in the refrigerator for at least an hour before serving.

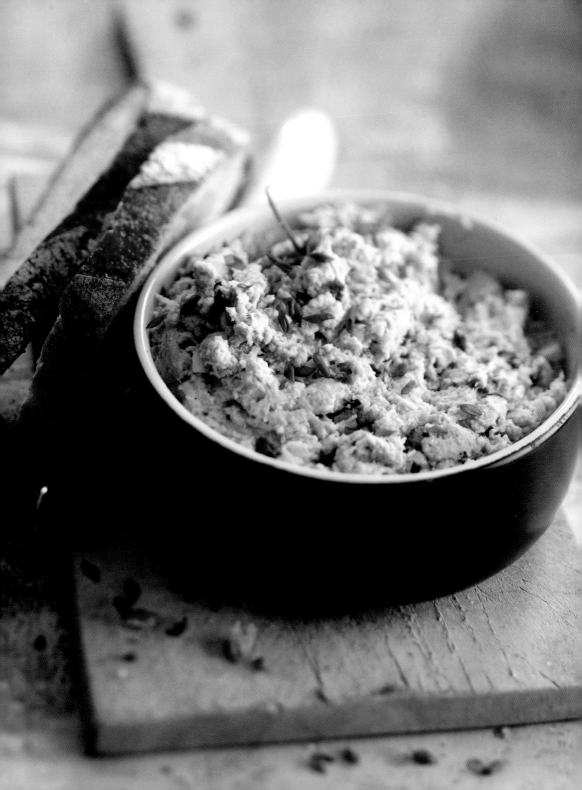

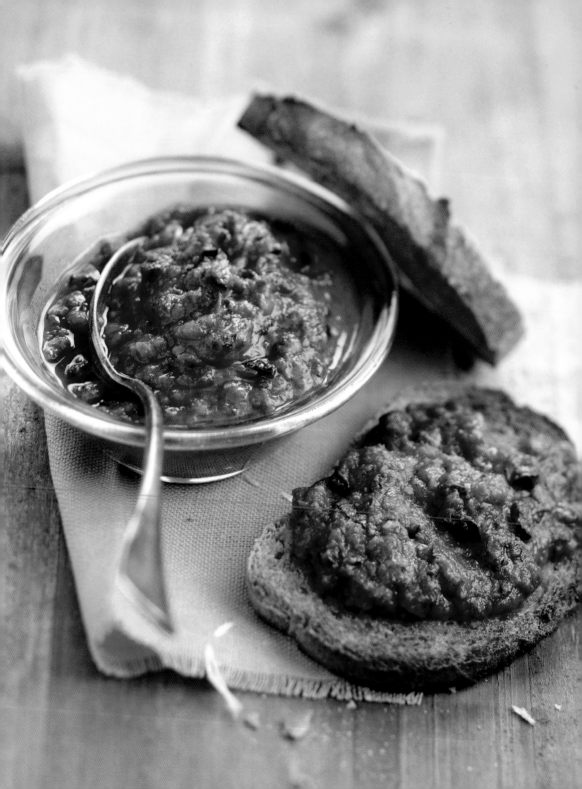

Tomato tapenade canapés
Toasts à la tapenade légère tomatée

It's easy to forget that olives are high in fat. So classic tapenade, which is made from olives, olive oil, and anchovies in oil, needs to be consumed in moderation. That's why we've come up with this low-fat recipe, which retains all the typical Mediterranean flavors of this dish.

PREP TIME 15 minutes

INGREDIENTS FOR 4 PEOPLE
4 thin slices (2 oz./60 g) wholegrain bread
12 fresh basil leaves
1 clove garlic
½ lemon
8 black olives, pitted
8 anchovy fillets without oil
½ teaspoon ground cumin
4 tablespoons crushed (chopped) tomatoes

1 Toast the slices of bread.

2 Rinse the basil leaves. Peel the garlic clove and squeeze the lemon.

3 Put the olives, anchovies, basil, lemon juice, garlic, and cumin into a food processor and process briefly. Stir in the crushed tomatoes and spread over the toasted bread.

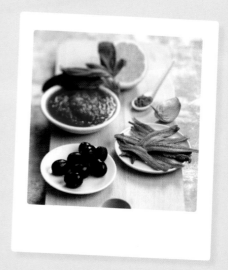

Tabbouleh
Taboulé

Tabbouleh is perfect for a picnic or to accompany meat grilled on the barbecue in summer. The version offered here is rich in vegetables and low in fat. Quick to prepare, it wins hands down against store-bought versions made from couscous with high-fat dressing and few vegetables.

PREP TIME 25 minutes | **COOK TIME** 15 minutes | **CHILL TIME** 1 hour 5 minutes

INGREDIENTS FOR 4 PEOPLE
½ cucumber (7 oz./200 g)
Scant 1 cup (7 oz./200 g) couscous
½ cup (3 ½ fl. oz./100 ml) lemon juice
1 ½ tablespoons chopped fresh mint
4 tomatoes
1 onion
4 teaspoons olive oil
4 pinches of finely chopped fresh basil or oregano
Salt and pepper

1 Wash, peel, and finely dice the cucumber. Put the couscous in a large mixing bowl and stir in ½ cup (3 ½ fl. oz./100 ml) water, the lemon juice, diced cucumber, and half the chopped mint. Refrigerate for 35 minutes.

2 Immerse the tomatoes in boiling water for a few seconds to loosen their skins, then peel, seed, and finely dice. Peel and finely chop the onion and put into a saucepan with the tomatoes, olive oil, and the remaining chopped fresh herbs. Cook over a low heat for about 15 minutes, until the tomatoes are no longer in pieces. Season with salt and pepper.

3 Add the tomato sauce to the couscous and mix well. Chill for an additional 30 minutes before serving.

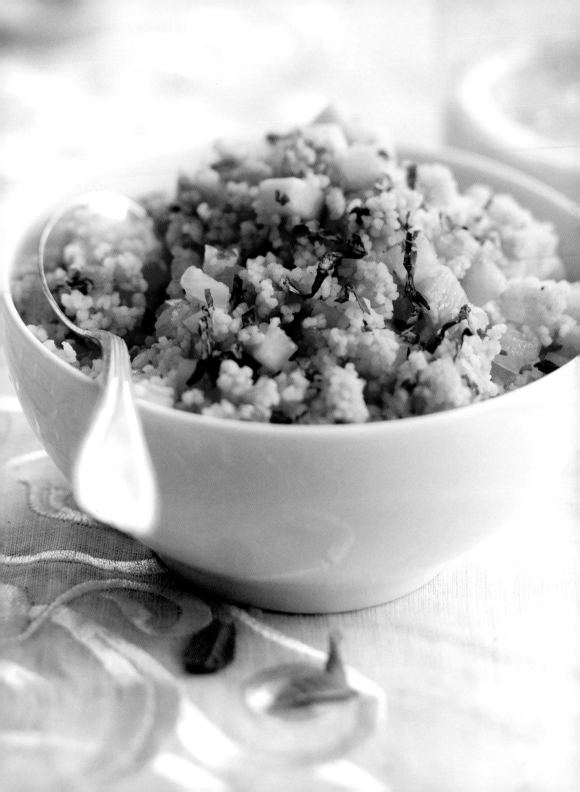

Chicken liver pâté
Pâté de foie de volaille

Commercial chicken liver pâté contains around 36 percent fat and yet liver is naturally low in lipids. It's therefore preferable to use this homemade recipe, which is made from chicken livers and nonfat petits-suisses (French cream cheese from Normandy; if unavailable, substitute fat-free cottage cheese and cream cheese) and thus is particularly low in calories.

PREP TIME 15 minutes | **COOK TIME** 10 minutes | **CHILL TIME** 8 hours

INGREDIENTS FOR 4 PEOPLE
2 shallots
1 lb. (500 g) chicken livers, cleaned and deveined
4 teaspoons brandy (optional)
1 small bunch parsley
8 plain nonfat petits-suisses, or generous ¾ cup (7 oz./200g)
   fat-free cottage cheese + scant ½ cup (4 oz./115 g) fat-free cream cheese
½ teaspoon grated nutmeg
Salt and pepper

1 Peel and chop the shallots and sauté with the chicken livers in a nonstick skillet (frying pan) without adding any fat.

2 Drain the petits-suisses (or cottage cheese) well. Put the chicken livers, shallots, parsley, petits-suisses (or cottage and cream cheeses), nutmeg, and salt and pepper into the bowl of a food processor and process until smooth.

3 Pack the pâté into a small terrine dish and refrigerate overnight.

Baked oysters
Huîtres gratinées

Oysters are the perfect diet food because they are naturally lean, containing only 1.2 percent fat. However, when you want a change from the traditional lemon juice or shallot vinegar, you'll find that alternative ways of serving oysters often seriously increase their calorific value. We propose this recipe for oven-baked oysters that is both very tasty and reasonably low in calories. This is a pleasure you don't need to resist!

PREP TIME 35 minutes | **COOK TIME** 20 minutes

INGREDIENTS FOR 4 PEOPLE
24 oysters
1 cup (½ pint/250 ml) dry white wine
   (preferably Muscadet)
1 tablespoon (½ oz./15 g) light butter, softened
2 tablespoons (⅓ oz./10 g) cornstarch (cornflour)

2 tablespoons low-fat sour cream
   (crème fraîche)
1 egg yolk
Pinch of cayenne pepper
2 tablespoons chopped parsley
Salt

1 Open the oysters and remove their flesh. Set aside the shells and pour the water from the oysters into a separate container. Strain this liquid and add white wine until you have 1 ¼ cups (10 fl. oz./300 ml) of liquid.

2 Preheat the oven to 450°F (230°C/Gas mark 8).

3 Put the oysters in a saucepan and cover with the white wine mixture. Cook over a low heat for 1–2 minutes, depending on the size of the oysters, but without the liquid reaching a simmer. Remove the oysters from the saucepan using a slotted spoon.

4 Reduce the liquid to about one third of its volume. In a small bowl, mix together the butter and cornstarch to make a beurre manié and add it to the liquid a little at a time, stirring constantly over a low heat, until the sauce becomes thick and smooth. Gradually stir in the sour cream. Remove from the heat and add the egg yolk, stirring constantly. Season with salt and cayenne pepper.

5 Choose the most attractive shells and wash and dry them. Place the shells open side up on a baking sheet, put an oyster in each one, and cover with a tablespoon of the sauce. Bake in the oven for about 10 minutes. Sprinkle over the chopped parsley and serve immediately.

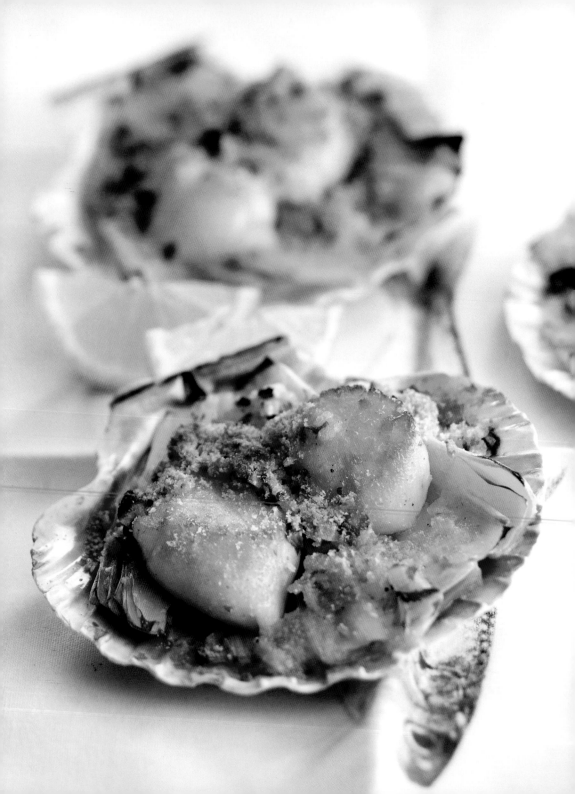

Breton-style scallops on a bed of leeks

Coquilles Saint-Jacques à la bretonne sur lit de poireaux

Scallops are lean seafood, but they are often cooked with excessive amounts of butter and cream. This recipe using low-fat sour cream (crème fraîche) remains low in calories and can easily feature on the menu for a special occasion without your guests suspecting that you're watching your weight.

PREP TIME 30 minutes | **COOK TIME** 1 hour

INGREDIENTS FOR 4 PEOPLE

14 oz. (400 g) leeks (white parts only)
4 shallots
20 scallops
½ bunch parsley
1 teaspoon fish stock

½ cup (4 ¼ fl. oz./125 ml) dry white wine
⅔ cup (5 fl. oz./150 ml) low-fat sour cream (crème fraîche)
2 crispbreads
Salt and pepper

1 Heat the broiler (grill).

2 Wash and trim the leeks and steam cook them until tender. Peel and finely chop the shallots. Using a sheet of paper towels, wipe the surface of a nonstick skillet (frying pan) with oil. Sear the scallops for 5 minutes on each side. Lay some chopped leeks in the bottom of four warmed shells or individual ovenproof dishes, then divide the scallops between them. In the same skillet, sauté the shallots until transparent. Wash and chop the parsley. Add it to the shallots and cook for an additional few minutes. Lower the heat.

3 Add the fish stock to the white wine and add to the pan. Stir in the sour cream and leave for 5 minutes. Add pepper and salt if necessary (bearing in mind that the fish stock is already salty).

4 Pour this sauce over the scallops. Crush the crispbreads with a mortar and pestle and divide between the shells or dishes.

5 Place under the broiler (grill) for a few minutes until golden brown on the top. Serve immediately.

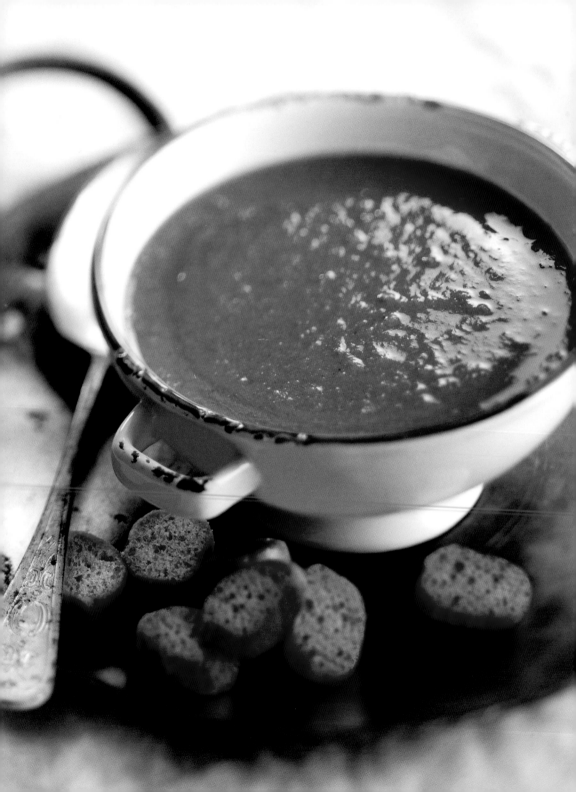

Fish soup
Soupe de poisson

A classic French dish, fish soup is often made with a substantial amount of oil and few of the best bits of fish, and thus contains little in the way of protein. This low-calorie version, however, is rich in flavor, proteins, and omega-3 fatty acids.

PREP TIME 35 minutes | **COOK TIME** 1 hour 15 minutes

INGREDIENTS FOR 4 PEOPLE

2 onions	1 medium rockfish
3 shallots	3 gurnard
3 cloves garlic	1 bouquet garni
1 lb. (500 g) fresh fish bones	A few fresh basil leaves
8 red mullet fillets	Juice of ½ lemon
A little flour for dusting the mullet fillets	4 tomatoes
	4 saffron threads
2 cans sardines in tomato sauce	4 pints (2 liters) fish stock
3 fresh whitings	¼ cup (1 ¾ oz./50 g) short-grain rice

1   Peel and finely chop the onions, shallots, and garlic, then dry-fry with the fish bones in a large cooking pot. Dust the red mullet fillets with flour, dry-fry them in a nonstick skillet (frying pan), then add them to the cooking pot along with the sardines. Clean the whiting, rockfish, and gurnard, remove their heads and fins, and cut them into pieces. Add to the pot with the bouquet garni, basil leaves, and lemon juice.

2   Cut the tomatoes into pieces and add them to the pot with the saffron threads and the fish stock. Add the rice and stir well to make sure it doesn't stick to the bottom of the pot. Simmer, covered, over a very low heat for about an hour.

3   Stir regularly to make sure that the fish doesn't stick to the bottom of the pot. When cooked, the fish bones will have turned soft and crumbly.

4   Pour the soup into a food processor or blender and liquidize. Pass the soup through a chinois (very fine sieve), pressing it with a small ladle to extract the maximum liquid (you should have about 4 pints/2 liters).

Beef and carrot stew
Bœuf-carottes diététique

This simple stew, in the style of the classic bœuf bourguignon, is a great family dish. Choose your piece of beef for braising carefully, avoiding the more fatty cuts. The wine sauce is slightly thickened with a little cornstarch (cornflour) rather than being made in the traditional way with lots of butter.

PREP TIME 30 minutes | **MARINATE TIME** 3 hours | **COOK TIME** 2 hours 15 minutes

INGREDIENTS FOR 4 PEOPLE
1 ¼ lb. (600 g) lean braising steak
1 ¾ lb. (800 g) carrots
1 or 2 cloves
⅔ cup (5 fl. oz./150 ml) red Burgundy wine
2 onions
2 tablespoons cornstarch (cornflour)
2 cloves garlic
1 bouquet garni
Salt, pepper, and peppercorns
Traditional wholegrain mustard, to serve (optional)

1 Cut the braising steak into large cubes. Wash, peel, and slice the carrots. Put the meat, carrots, cloves, and some peppercorns into a dish and pour over the wine. Let marinate in the refrigerator for at least 3 hours.

2 Peel and finely chop the onions and dry-fry them in a nonstick cooking pot. Drain the marinated meat (reserving the marinade) and add to the pot. Sprinkle over the cornstarch, stir to coat the meat, and brown the meat over a high heat. Peel and crush the garlic and add to the pot, pour over the marinade, and stir well, topping up with a little water if necessary. Season with salt and pepper and add the bouquet garni.

3 Simmer, covered, for 1 ½ hours over a low heat, then add the carrots and continue to cook for an additional 30 minutes.

4 Serve hot with traditional wholegrain mustard.

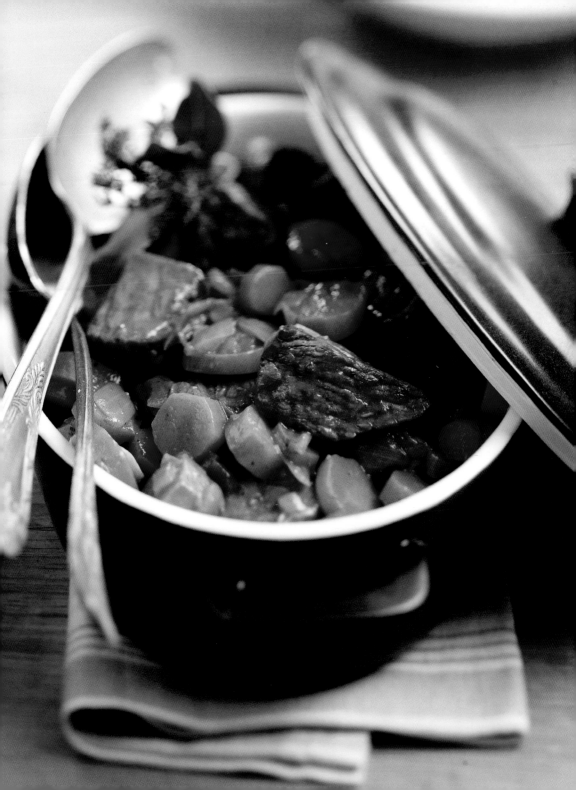

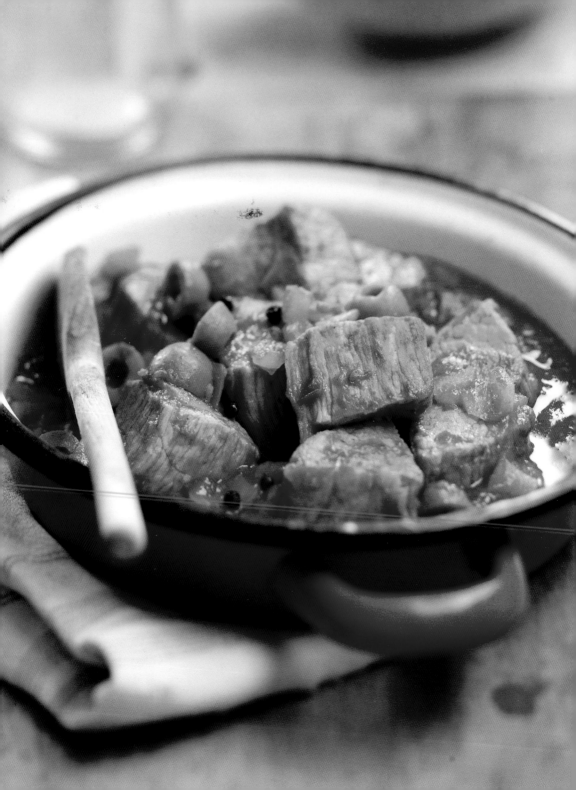

Sautéed veal with olives
Sauté de veau léger aux olives

People often avoid meat cooked with sauce when they're watching their weight, but that's not really necessary. By choosing a lean cut of meat and removing any visible fat, as in this veal stew, and by replacing the butter that's often used in cooking such dishes and their sauces with a tomato and green olive sauce, you can have an easy meat recipe with a healthy sauce that's rich in antioxidants.

PREP TIME 20 minutes | **COOK TIME** 1 hour

INGREDIENTS FOR 4 PEOPLE
2 onions
1 lb. (500 g) lean stewing veal
1 tablespoon sunflower oil
3 teaspoons tomato paste (purée)
16 green olives, pitted
15-oz. (425-g) can crushed (chopped) tomatoes
Salt and pepper

1   Peel and finely chop the onions and cut the veal into cubes. Heat the oil in a nonstick sauté pan and brown the meat. Add the onions. Continue to cook for an additional 3 minutes.

2   Dissolve the tomato paste in 1 ⅔ cups (13 ½ fl. oz./400 ml) water and pour over the meat. Slice the olives and add them to the pan. Season with salt and pepper and let simmer for 30 minutes.

3   Add the crushed tomatoes and cook for an additional 20 minutes.

4   Serve hot.

Buckwheat pancakes with mushrooms

Galettes de sarrasin aux champignons

The Breton buckwheat pancake (galette au sarrasin) is very healthy as it contains simply buckwheat flour, water, eggs, and salt. It's the filling and the amount of fat used for cooking that modify its calorific value. If you choose lean, nutritional ingredients, such as lean ham and eggs, and enrich it with vegetables, such as sautéed mushrooms, you'll have a quick, simple, and balanced meal for all the family.

PREP TIME 25 minutes | **COOK TIME** 30 minutes

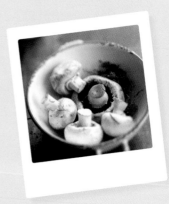

INGREDIENTS FOR 4 PEOPLE
2 onions
1 ¾ lb. (800 g) mushrooms
2 slices good-quality lean ham
4 buckwheat pancakes (ready-made
   or packet mix)
4 eggs
A few fresh chives
Salt and pepper

1 Preheat the oven to 350°F (180°C/Gas mark 4).

2 Peel and finely chop the onions and dry-fry them in a nonstick skillet (frying pan). Clean the mushrooms with damp paper towels, then dice the caps and stalks and add them to the onions. Continue to cook until the mushrooms have turned golden.

3 Lay half a slice of ham in the center of each pancake, add the mushrooms, and fold over the edges to form a square package. Cook in the oven on a baking sheet covered with parchment (greaseproof) paper for 20 minutes.

4 Wipe the skillet with a little oil on some paper towels and fry the eggs. Season with salt and sprinkle with a few chopped chives.

5 Serve the pancakes hot, topped with a fried egg.

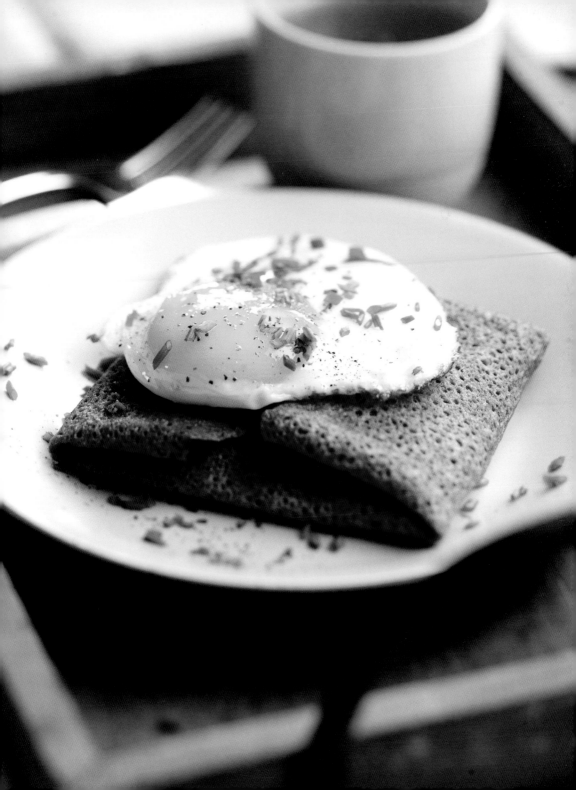

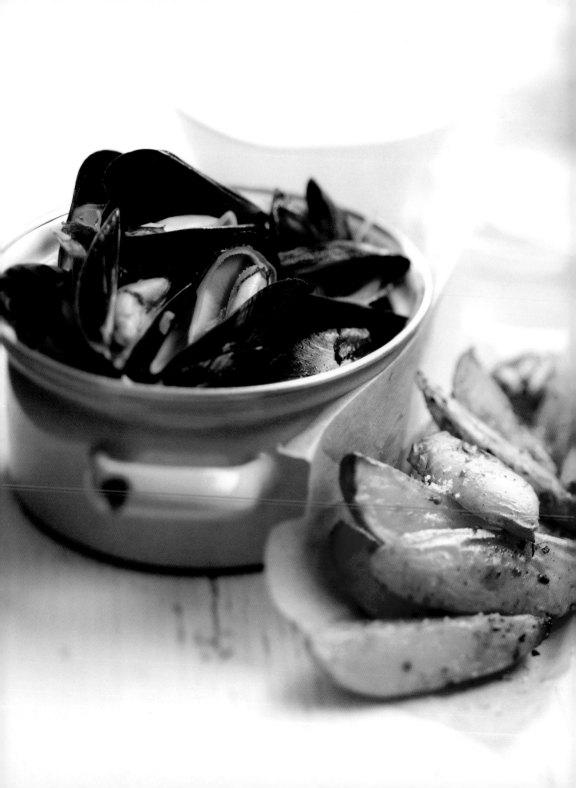

Moules marinières
with potato wedges

What would mussels be without the accompaniment of crispy fries? The classic moules-frites combination can be made healthy if you cook the potatoes in the oven instead of immersing them in oil. Change your habits and discover the secret of light fries.

PREP TIME 35 minutes | **MARINATE TIME** 30 minutes | **COOK TIME** 35 minutes

INGREDIENTS FOR 4 PEOPLE
14 oz. (400 g) potatoes
1 clove garlic
2 teaspoons paprika
4 teaspoons thyme leaves
Juice of ½ lemon
1 tablespoon olive oil
8 ½ pints or 7 lb. (4 liters or 3.2 kg)
    mussels in shells
½ onion
1 small bunch parsley
½ cup (4 ¼ fl. oz./125 ml) dry white wine
Salt and pepper

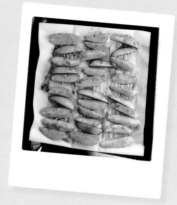

1 Preheat the oven to 400°F (200°C/Gas mark 6).

2 Wash and scrub the potatoes and cut them in quarters lengthwise without peeling them. Peel and finely chop the garlic clove. In a large bowl, mix together the garlic, paprika, thyme, lemon juice, olive oil, salt, and pepper, then add the potato wedges and turn to coat thoroughly. Let marinate for 30 minutes.

3 Spread out the potato wedges and their marinade on a baking sheet covered with parchment (greaseproof) paper, making sure they are well spaced out. Cook in the oven for 30 minutes, turning them over halfway through the cooking time. Prepare the mussels. Scrub them under running water and pull off the little "beards."

4 Peel and finely chop the onion and dry-fry in a nonstick cooking pot large enough to hold the mussels. Chop the parsley and add to the pot with the white wine. Add the mussels and cook, stirring, until all the mussels are open. Discard any that stay closed.

5 Serve the mussels hot with the potato wedges.

Sauerkraut
Choucroute minceur

A truly iconic dish from Alsace, sauerkraut has quite a history. Easy to conserve and rich in vitamin C, it has long helped in the fight against scurvy among sailors on lengthy voyages and in improving the health of the local population during winter. Sauerkraut, without its accompaniment, is particularly healthy and plays a beneficial role in digestion. If you take the trouble to cook it yourself and to accompany it with lean cuts of meat, this is an easy dish that you can enjoy at any time of year.

PREP TIME 25 minutes | **COOK TIME** 2 hours 10 minutes

INGREDIENTS FOR 4 PEOPLE
Generous ¾ cup (7 oz./200 g) raw sauerkraut (available from health
    food stores and farmers' markets)
1 onion
1 bunch parsley
4 teaspoons juniper berries
½ cup (¼ pint/125 ml) dry white wine (ideally from Alsace)
1-lb. (500-g) knuckle of pork (not breaded), trimmed of visible fat
4 slices lean ham
4 small chicken sausages
Salt and pepper

1 Bring a pot of water to a boil, drain the sauerkraut and add to the boiling water, and cook for 10 minutes. Drain and rinse. Repeat the cooking process once more.

2 Peel and finely chop the onion and dry-fry in a nonstick cooking pot. Wash, dry, and chop the parsley, and add to the pot with the juniper berries, then add the white wine. Add the sauerkraut, season with salt and pepper, then fill the pot to half full with water, and cook over a low heat, covered, for 1 ½ hours, stirring occasionally.

3 Lay the pork knuckle, rolled-up slices of ham, and chicken sausages on top of the sauerkraut, cover and cook for an additional 15 minutes.

4 Serve hot.

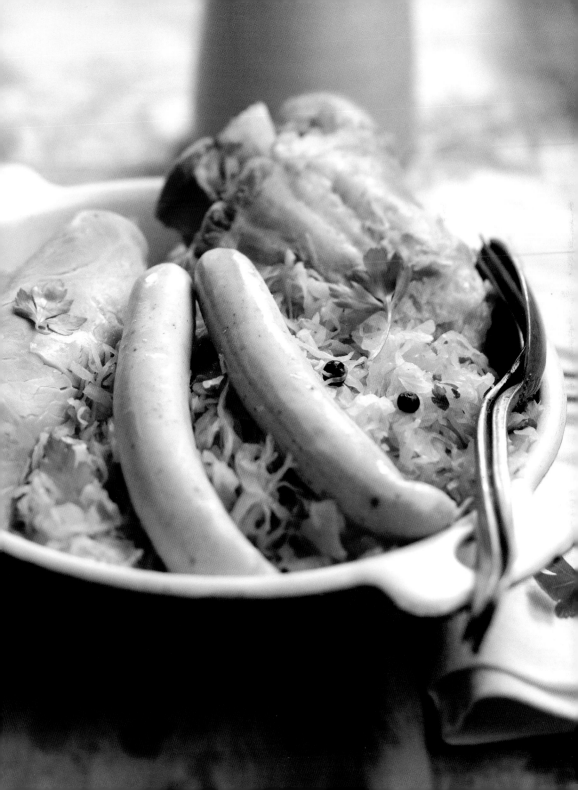

Orloff-style veal skewers with onions

Brochettes de veau façon orloff à la fondue d'oignons

Veal is one of the leanest white meats, particularly cutlets. Here it is prepared like Veal Orloff, but the cooked cheese (Parmesan, Comté, Emmental), which is high in fats, is replaced with cheese slices. Choosing slices of lean Canadian (back) bacon as opposed to streaky bacon also reduces the amount of fat while preserving the original taste of this dish, with melted cheese, the aroma of bacon and, to accompany it, sautéed onions rather than the traditional cheese sauce.

PREP TIME 30 minutes | **COOK TIME** 25 minutes

INGREDIENTS FOR 4 PEOPLE
2 onions
4 veal cutlets (4 oz./115 g each)
8 slices of Canadian-style (back) bacon
4 cheese slices (¾ oz./20 g per slice)
4 teaspoons thyme leaves
Salt and pepper

1 Preheat the oven to 350°F (180°C/Gas mark 4).

2 Peel and chop the onions and dry-fry them in a nonstick skillet (frying pan) until they are golden brown. Add a glass of water, salt, and pepper, and continue to cook over a low heat until the onions have completely softened.

3 Cut the veal cutlets, bacon, and cheese slices into strips about ¾ in. (2 cm) wide. Layer a piece of veal, a strip of bacon, and a strip of cheese slice and roll up. Thread these rolls onto skewers and sprinkle with thyme.

4 Place the skewers on a baking sheet covered with a sheet of parchment (greaseproof) paper and cook in the oven for 10 minutes. Finish under the broiler (grill).

5 Serve hot with the onions.

Provençal fish and vegetables with aioli garlic mayonnaise
Le grand aïoli, sauce légère à l'ail

This famous Provençal sauce is in fact mayonnaise made from olive oil, egg yolks, and crushed raw garlic, usually without mustard. You no doubt know of light mayonnaise: now discover light aioli!

PREP TIME 30 minutes | **COOK TIME** 35 minutes | **CHILL TIME** 10 minutes

INGREDIENTS FOR 4 PEOPLE
14 oz. (400 g) cauliflower
14 oz. (400 g) green beans
14 oz. (400 g) carrots
14 oz. (400 g) potatoes
1 ¼ lb. (600 g) cooked whelks
2 tablespoons vegetable bouillon powder
1 lb. (500 g) cod fillets

FOR THE SAUCE
1 egg
2 cloves garlic
2 teaspoons mustard
2 plain nonfat petits-suisses, or 7 tablespoons
  (3 ½ oz./100 g) fat-free cottage cheese
1 ¼ cups (10 ½ oz./300 g) nonfat fromage
  blanc or plain nonfat regular or Greek yogurt
Salt and pepper

1 Wash and peel the vegetables and steam cook them until tender but still crisp to the bite.

2 Arrange the vegetables around the edge of a large serving plate and place the whelks in the center.

3 Dissolve the vegetable bouillon powder in 4 cups (2 pints/1 liter) of boiling water and poach the cod fillets at a simmer for 5–10 minutes until just cooked through. Drain the cod, let cool, and arrange alongside the whelks in the center of the plate.

4 Prepare the light garlic mayonnaise. Hard-boil the egg. Drain the petits-suisses (or cottage cheese) well. Peel and crush the garlic cloves into a bowl. Mash the egg with the mustard, crushed garlic, and the petits-suisses (or cottage cheese). Season with salt and pepper and stir in the fromage blanc or yogurt. Refrigerate until ready to serve.

5 Serve the plate of fish and vegetables with the light garlic mayonnaise.

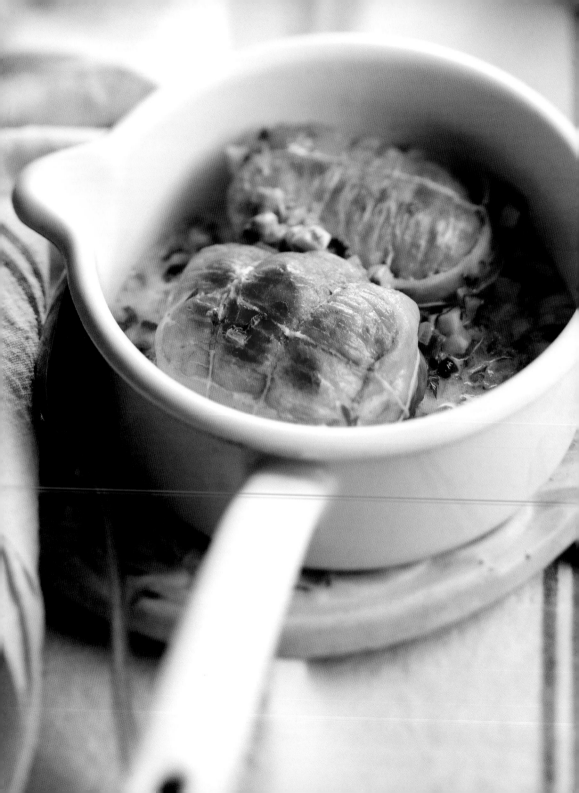

Veal paupiettes with mushrooms

Paupiettes de veau aux champignons

The thin slice of veal used to make paupiettes is usually of good nutritional value, but it's the stuffing that can lighten (or increase) the calorific value of the dish. The stuffing used in this recipe, made from ham and lean pork, is high in quality and low in fat.

PREP TIME 40 minutes | **COOK TIME** 40 minutes

INGREDIENTS FOR 4 PEOPLE

4 veal cutlets	1 ¼ cups (10 fl. oz./300 ml) veal stock
1 onion	7 oz. (200 g) mushrooms
2 shallots	1 tablespoon chopped parsley
4 ½ oz. (125 g) lean ham	4 tablespoons low-fat (3% fat) sour
3 ½ oz. (100 g) lean pork	cream (crème fraîche)
tenderloin (fillet)	Salt and pepper

1 Flatten the veal cutlets using a meat mallet (or a rolling pin) so that they are very thin. Trim them to give them a regular shape. Peel and finely chop the onion and one of the shallots. Finely chop the ham, pork, and the offcuts of veal. Mix the chopped meats, onion, and shallot in a bowl and season with salt and pepper.

2 Place a quarter of this stuffing mixture at one end of a veal cutlet and roll up the cutlet around the filling. Tie up the paupiette with a length of kitchen string. Repeat to make three more paupiettes.

3 Heat a nonstick sauté pan and brown the paupiettes on each side. Pour over the stock, cover the pan, and simmer over a low heat for 30 minutes.

4 Remove and discard the end of the mushroom stalks, then wipe and finely chop the mushrooms. Peel and finely chop the remaining shallot. Dry-fry the shallot in a small nonstick skillet (frying pan) over a high heat for 3 minutes. Add the mushrooms and cook, stirring, for 10 minutes, until there is no more liquid. Add the chopped parsley, salt, and pepper.

5 When the paupiettes are cooked, remove from the pan with a slotted spoon and keep warm, then reduce the stock and stir in the mushroom and shallot mixture. Remove the pan from the heat and stir in the cream. Heat until just simmering, and serve immediately with the paupiettes.

Pot-au-feu

This traditional French dish of boiled beef is renowned for its long cooking time over a very low heat in a broth flavored with vegetables and a bouquet garni. The calorific value of this recipe has been reduced by the careful choice of meat and by cooking without any fat.

PREP TIME 35 minutes | **COOK TIME** 50 minutes

INGREDIENTS FOR 4 PEOPLE

6 small carrots
4 small turnips
2 onions
1 celery stick
3 leeks
1 clove garlic
2 teaspoons kosher (sea) salt
1 bouquet garni
1 teaspoon peppercorns

3 cloves
1 ¾ lb. (800 g) beef shank (shin)
2 skinless chicken thighs (6 ½ oz./180 g
    total)
8 small potatoes
½ lemon
1 marrowbone
Kosher salt, pickles (pickled gherkins),
    and mustard, to serve (optional)

1   Peel the carrots, turnips, onions, and celery, and trim and wash the leeks and celery. Cut the leeks in half and stick the cloves into the onions. Peel and crush the garlic.

2   Pour about 4 pints (2 liters) of water into a pressure cooker and add the salt, bouquet garni, peppercorns, and all of the vegetables prepared above. Bring to a boil. When the water begins to boil, add the piece of beef and the chicken thighs. Close the lid of the pressure cooker and bring up to pressure over a high heat. Once the valve begins to whistle, reduce the heat and cook for 35 minutes over a low heat.

3   Scrub the potatoes. Squeeze lemon juice over the ends of the marrowbone and add to the pressure cooker with the potatoes. Replace the lid and continue to cook over a low heat for an additional 15 minutes.

4   Serve a piece of each meat surrounded by the different vegetables and two potatoes per person. Pass around kosher salt, pickles, mustard, and a small bowl of the stock for people to help themselves. You can finish off the tasty stock the next day, but cool it completely so that you can skim it of any fat before reheating it.

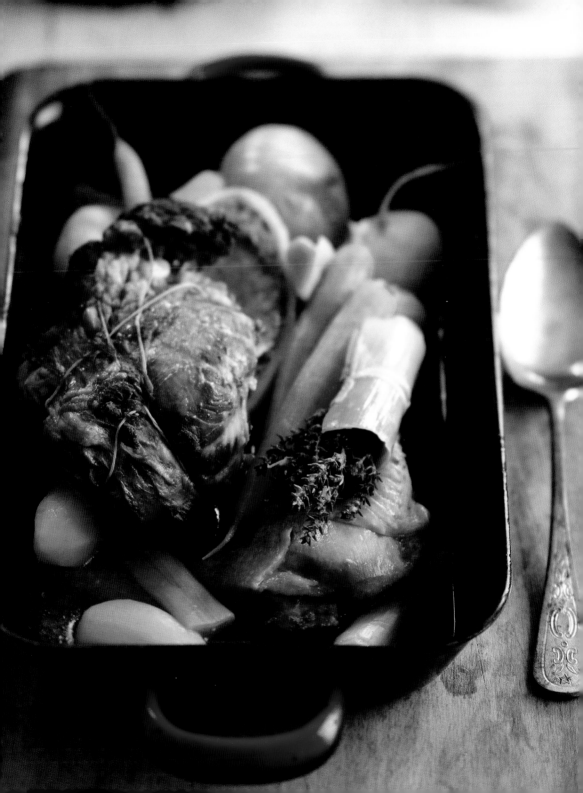

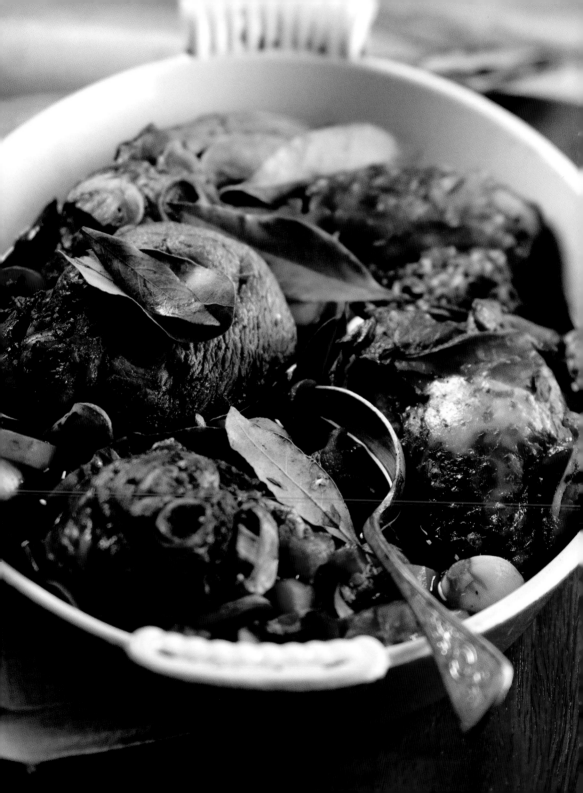

Coq au vin

This is a classic of French gastronomy that lovers of French food will definitely want to include in a weight-loss diet! Traditionally made with cock, many recipes use chicken which is more readily available. Here, the chicken is covered with lean bacon and the marinade is low-calorie.

PREP TIME 45 minutes | **MARINATE TIME** 24 hours | **COOK TIME** 1 hour 50 minutes

INGREDIENTS FOR 4 PEOPLE
1 x 4-lb. (1.8-kg) chicken
2 carrots
2 onions
2 cloves garlic
3 ½ oz. (100 g) lean smoked Canadian-
    style (back) bacon, finely chopped
1 bouquet garni
9 oz. (250 g) button mushrooms
16 pearl onions
Salt and pepper

FOR THE MARINADE
2 carrots
2 cloves garlic
2 large onions
1 bunch parsley
1 teaspoon peppercorns
2 bay leaves
1 sprig thyme
6 cups (3 pints/1.5 liters) red wine

1   Prepare the marinade: peel, wash, and slice the carrots. Peel and crush the garlic. Peel and finely chop the onions. Put them in a large dish and add the parsley, peppercorns, bay leaves, and thyme. Cut the chicken into pieces. Place them in the dish, pour over the wine, cover, and let marinate in the refrigerator for 24 hours.

2   Drain the pieces of chicken and pat them dry. Strain the marinade and reserve the liquid. Peel, wash, and slice the carrots. Peel and finely chop the onions (but not the pearl onions). Peel and crush the garlic. Preheat the oven to 300°F (150°C/Gas mark 2).

3   Brown the chicken pieces on all sides in a cooking pot without adding any fat. Set aside. In the same pot, brown the chopped bacon, chopped onions, and sliced carrots. Remove from the pot and set aside. Remove any fat from the pot, then return the vegetables, bacon, and chicken pieces to the pot and add the bouquet garni and crushed garlic. Season with salt and pepper. Pour over the reserved marinade and slowly bring to a boil. Cover the pot and place in the oven for 1 hour.

4   Remove and discard the end of the mushroom stalks, then wipe the mushrooms. Peel the pearl onions. Add the whole mushrooms and pearl onions to the pot, return to the oven, and cook for an additional 30 minutes. Check that the chicken is cooked: the pieces should be tender. If there is too much juice, remove the chicken pieces and heat the liquid to reduce it.

Fondue bourguignonne

Fondue bourguignonne is high in calories for two reasons: firstly, the meat is cooked in oil, and secondly, it is accompanied by high-fat sauces. To reduce its calorific value, cook the meat in stock and make tasty, low-calorie sauces, which will flavor the meat wonderfully.

INGREDIENTS FOR 4 PEOPLE
1 ¼ lb. (600 g) lean beef
4 pints (2 liters) beef stock (made with 4 beef bouillon cubes)

1 Cut the meat into small pieces and place in a dish. Make the different sauces (see recipes below).

2 Pour the hot stock into the fondue pot. Guests can then skewer a piece of meat and cook it in the stock before eating it with sauces of their choice: mustard, reduced-sugar ketchup, or homemade sauces (see below).

Tomato chutney

PREP TIME 15 minutes | **COOK TIME** 15 minutes

INGREDIENTS FOR 4 PEOPLE

3 very ripe tomatoes
1 apple
2 cloves garlic
1 teaspoon traditional wholegrain mustard
½ teaspoon ground coriander
½ teaspoon ground ginger

Pinch of mild chili powder
Scant ½ cup (3 ½ fl. oz./100 ml) balsamic vinegar
3 tablespoons (1oz./30 g) raisins
Salt

1 Peel, seed, and cut the tomatoes and apple into small pieces. Peel and crush the garlic cloves.

2 In a small saucepan, heat the mustard, spices, vinegar, and garlic for a few seconds, then add the tomatoes, apple, and the raisins. Season with salt. Stir together and cook over a medium heat for 10 minutes.

Caper sauce

PREP TIME 10 minutes | **CHILL TIME** 15 minutes

INGREDIENTS FOR 4 PEOPLE
1 onion, finely chopped
Juice of 1 lemon
2 cups (1 lb./480 g) nonfat fromage blanc or plain nonfat regular or Greek yogurt
20 capers
Salt and pepper

1 Stir all the ingredients together in a bowl.

2 Refrigerate until ready to serve.

Barbecue sauce

PREP TIME 15 minutes | **COOK TIME** 25 minutes

INGREDIENTS FOR 4 PEOPLE
14 oz. (400 g) tomatoes
2 onions
4 cloves garlic
4 pinches of cayenne pepper
2 teaspoons tomato paste (purée)
Salt

1 Peel, seed, and dice the tomatoes. Peel and finely chop the onions and garlic.

2 Dry-fry the onions and garlic in a nonstick skillet (frying pan), then add the diced tomatoes and a glass of water. Season with salt and the cayenne pepper and stir in the tomato paste. Reduce the sauce over a low heat for 15 minutes.

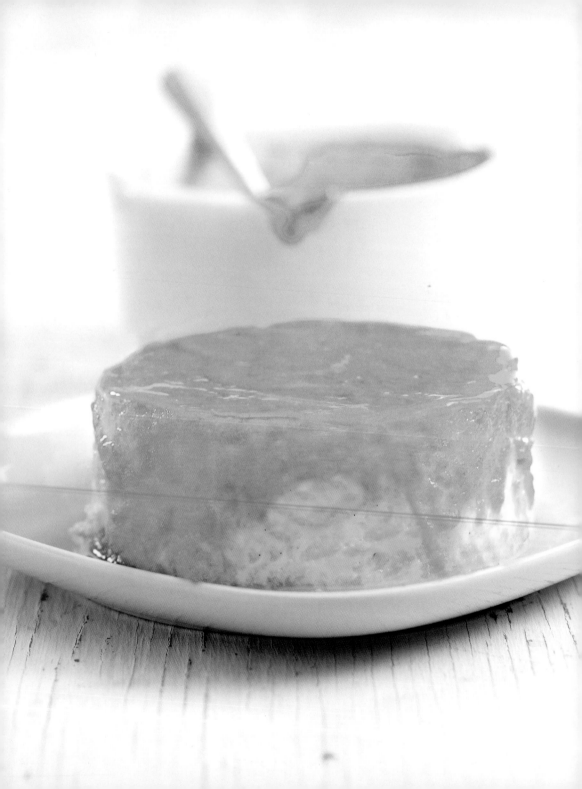

Baked rice pudding with exotic fruit coulis

Gâteau de riz au coulis de fruits exotiques

This dessert is traditionally a vanilla-flavored rice pudding bound with eggs on a caramel base, which is baked in the oven. Made with fat-free milk and topped with a coulis of exotic fruits, this version is a dessert you can indulge in with peace of mind.

PREP TIME 15 minutes | **FREEZE TIME** 20 minutes | **COOK TIME** 1 hour 15 minutes

INGREDIENTS FOR 4 PEOPLE

4 ¼ cups (2 pints/1 liter) fat-free milk
½ vanilla bean (pod)
½ cup (3 ½ oz./100 g) short-grain (pudding) rice
4 teaspoons powdered sweetener for cooking
4 tablespoons exotic fruit coulis (if unavailable,
    make your own using 1 ripe mango [5 oz./140 g] + juice of ½ lemon +
    2 tablespoons water)
2 eggs

1 Preheat the oven to 350°F (180°C/Gas mark 4).

2 Pour the milk into a saucepan. Split and scrape the vanilla bean, then stir the seeds into the milk. Bring to a boil, then pour in the rice and cook over a low heat for 30 minutes. Remove from the heat, stir in the sweetener, and let cool down to lukewarm.

3 If making your own fruit coulis, peel the mango, remove the flesh, and cut into small pieces. Place in a food processor or blender with the lemon juice and water and liquidize until a very smooth coulis is obtained. If necessary, add a little sweetener to taste. Pour 4 tablespoons of exotic fruit coulis into the bottom of a charlotte mold and put it in the freezer.

4 In a mixing bowl, beat the eggs, then slowly pour over the lukewarm rice and milk, stirring constantly. Let cool completely.

5 Remove the charlotte mold from the freezer and pour the cooled rice mixture over the top of the solidified coulis. Bake in the oven in a bain-marie for 30–35 minutes.

6 Remove the baked rice pudding from the oven and turn it out onto a plate. Serve either warm or cold, depending on your taste.

Coconut macaroons
Rochers coco légers

These little coconut cakes are very sweet petits-fours made with eggs and shredded (desiccated) coconut. This simple recipe made using sweetener will satisfy all the family while allowing you to economize on calories.

PREP TIME 15 minutes | **COOK TIME** 15 minutes

INGREDIENTS FOR 4 PEOPLE
4 tablespoons shredded (desiccated) coconut
2 tablespoons powdered sweetener for cooking
2 tablespoons cornstarch (cornflour)
1 egg
Pinch of salt

1 Preheat the oven to 350°F (180°C/Gas mark 4).

2 Mix all the ingredients together in a bowl.

3 Form little balls of the mixture on a baking sheet covered with parchment (greaseproof) paper and bake in the oven for 10–15 minutes until golden.

4 Let cool before eating.

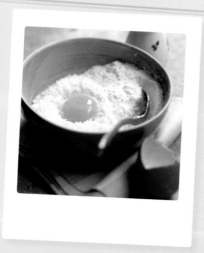
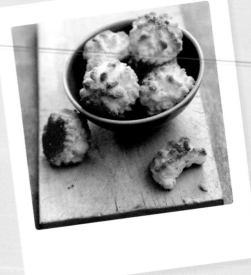

Breton *Far* with prunes
Far breton léger aux pruneaux

Far is a traditional recipe from Brittany and the most famous variation contains prunes. Enjoy this creamy yet low-fat version in which vanilla sugar is replaced by a vanilla bean for a more flavorsome dessert.

PREP TIME 20 minutes | **COOK TIME** 30 minutes

INGREDIENTS FOR 4 PEOPLE
1 ¼ cups (5 oz./150 g) cake (soft white) flour
4 tablespoons powdered sweetener for cooking
3 eggs
½ vanilla bean (pod)
2 ½ cups (1 ¼ pints/600 ml) fat-free milk
3 oz. (80 g) pitted prunes

1   Preheat the oven to 400°F (200°C/Gas mark 6).

2   In a bowl, mix all but 1 tablespoon of the flour with the sweetener and eggs until you obtain a smooth batter.

3   Split the vanilla bean and add the seeds to the mixture, then gradually pour in the milk, continuing to mix as you do so.

4   Line an ovenproof dish with parchment (grease-proof) paper and tip in the prunes. Add the remaining tablespoon of flour, turn the prunes to ensure they are well coated in flour, and spread them out in the base of the dish. Pour over the batter and bake in the oven for about 30 minutes.

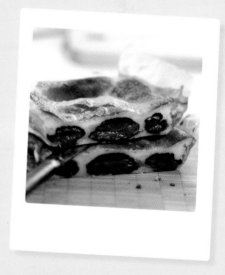

Almond cream–filled dates and prunes
Fruits déguisés à la farce amandine légère

"Disguised fruits," as their French name translates, are little treats made from dried fruit filled with colored marzipan. They are often served as part of the "thirteen desserts" that are traditional Christmastime fare in Provence. Impress your guests by making them with this delicious almond filling made with vanilla-flavored light cream mixed with just the right amount of ground almonds—a saving in calories that detracts nothing from the flavors of these delicacies.

PREP TIME 25 minutes | **COOK TIME** 25 minutes | **CHILL TIME** 2 hours

INGREDIENTS FOR 4 PEOPLE
¼ cup (1 ¼ oz./35 g) cornstarch (cornflour)
1 ⅔ cups (13 ½ fl. oz./400 ml) fat-free milk
½ vanilla bean (pod)
8 teaspoons powdered sweetener for cooking
Scant ¾ cup (2 oz./60 g) finely ground blanched almonds
A few drops of pink and green food coloring
2 oz. (60 g) pitted prunes
2 oz. (60 g) pitted dried dates

1 Dissolve the cornstarch in a scant ½ cup (3 ½ fl. oz./100 ml) of cold milk. Heat the remaining 1 ¼ cups (10 fl. oz./300 ml) of milk in a small saucepan with the split and scraped vanilla bean and let infuse for a few minutes.

2 Remove the vanilla bean from the milk, add the dissolved cornstarch and 4 teaspoons of sweetener, and heat over a low heat until you have a thick cream. Sprinkle in the ground almonds, mix in well, and divide between two bowls.

3 Add a few drops of pink food coloring to one bowl and a few drops of green coloring to the other. Stir well and refrigerate for 2 hours.

4 Cut slits in the dried fruits using a sharp knife. Remove the almond creams from the refrigerator and use to fill the fruits. Sprinkle the remaining sweetener onto a plate and roll each fruit in it to coat. Serve immediately.

Chocolate cookies
Merveilles au chocolat

Meringues are the least calorific of all cakes, which is why we have used them for the basis of this crisp cookie. We've also created a healthy version of chocolate cream with reduced-calorie ingredients.

PREP TIME 35 minutes | **CHILL TIME** 30 minutes | **COOK TIME** 40 minutes

INGREDIENTS FOR 4 COOKIES

Scant 1 tablespoon flour + a little for dusting the mold

2 tablespoons (⅓ oz./10 g) cornstarch (cornflour)

⅓ cup (1 oz./25 g) finely ground blanched almonds

4 tablespoons powdered sweetener for cooking

3 ½ tablespoons (1 ½ oz./40 g) superfine (caster) sugar

¼ stick (1 oz./25 g) light butter + a little for greasing the mold

2 egg whites

FOR THE CREAM

3 ½ oz. (100 g) dark (unsweetened) chocolate

½ cup (¼ pint/125 ml) light half-and-half (single cream)

2 ½ tablespoons (1 ¼ oz./35 g) light butter, softened

¼ cup (1 ¾ oz./50 g) chocolate sprinkles

1   Preheat the oven to 325°F (160°C/Gas mark 3).

2   In a bowl, mix together the flour, cornstarch, ground almonds, sweetener, and 1 ½ tablespoons of sugar. Melt the butter and set aside. Whisk the egg whites until they begin to thicken, then add the remaining 2 tablespoons of sugar and continue to whisk until firm. Pour the whisked egg whites over the almond mixture and fold in gently. Carefully stir in the melted butter. Lightly grease and dust with flour four individual ramekins. Divide the mixture between the ramekins and bake in the oven for 15–20 minutes.

3   Break the chocolate into small pieces. Pour the cream into a small saucepan and bring to a boil. Remove the pan from the heat and stir in the chocolate. Let stand for 2 minutes then stir with a spatula and let cool slightly. Cut the butter into small pieces and whisk into the chocolate cream. It should be smooth and creamy. Refrigerate for 30 minutes.

4   Turn the cookies out of the ramekins and cut each one in two horizontally. Spread a little of the chocolate cream on one half and top with the second. Cover the tops of the cookies with the rest of the cream (reheated if necessary) then dust with the chocolate sprinkles. Refrigerate the cookies until ready to serve.

Crème brûlée with a crisp fruity topping
Crème brûlée allégée en croûte rouge

Crème brûlée is a variation of the Spanish crema catalana. Traditionally made from egg yolks, sugar, and cream, it is high in fat and calories. So that you can continue to enjoy it, the ingredients have been lightened here, but not the taste, which is enhanced with a crisp fruity topping.

PREP TIME 15 minutes | **COOK TIME** 1 hour 10 minutes | **CHILL TIME** 1 hour 30 minutes

INGREDIENTS FOR 4 PEOPLE

3 egg yolks

1 tablespoon vanilla sugar (if unavailable, make your own using 1 vanilla bean to 2 cups (14 oz./400 g) granulated sugar*)

3 tablespoons powdered sweetener for cooking

1 ¼ cups (10 fl. oz./300 ml) light half-and-half (single cream)

Scant ½ cup (3 ½ fl. oz./100 ml) fat-free milk

4 tablespoons red berry coulis (if unavailable, make your own using 2 cups (8 oz./225 g) assorted red berries + 2 tablespoons water)

1 Preheat the oven to 225°F (110°C/Gas mark ¼).

2 In a bowl, mix together the egg yolks, vanilla sugar, sweetener, cream, and milk. Divide the mixture between four ramekins, place in a bain-marie and cook in the oven for 1 hour, until set. Remove from the oven, let cool, then refrigerate for 1 ½ hours.

3 Just before serving, heat the broiler (grill).

4 If making your own coulis, place the berries in a food processor or blender with the water and liquidize until a very smooth coulis is obtained. Strain through a chinois (fine sieve) to remove any seeds. If necessary, add a little sweetener to taste. Pour 4 tablespoons of coulis into a small saucepan and heat until reduced by half. Remove the crèmes brûlées from the refrigerator and pour over the fruit coulis, spreading it with the back of a spoon. Place the crèmes brûlées under the broiler (grill) for a few minutes, keeping a careful eye on them until the coulis forms a thin, red caramelized crust.

* To make your own vanilla sugar, slit the vanilla bean and scrape out the seeds into the sugar. Mix well or process in a food processor to make sure the seeds are evenly distributed throughout the sugar. Store in an airtight container with the scraped-out pod for 1–2 weeks before using.

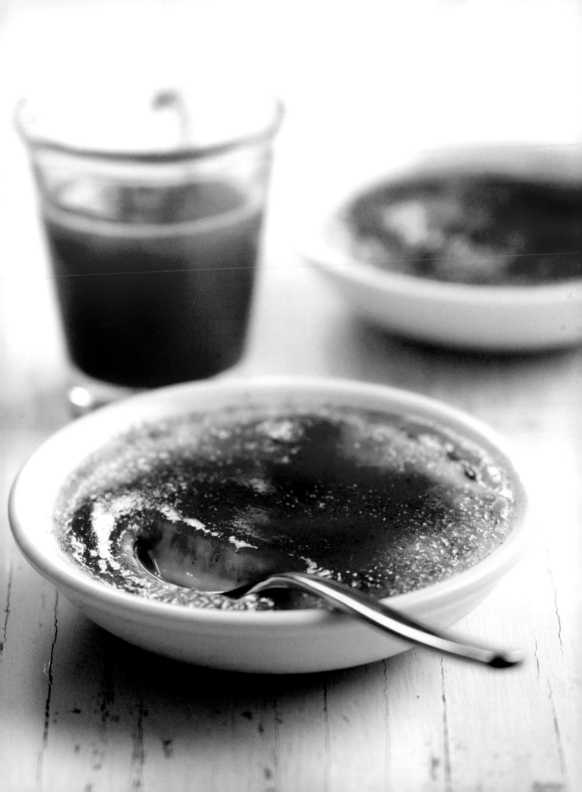

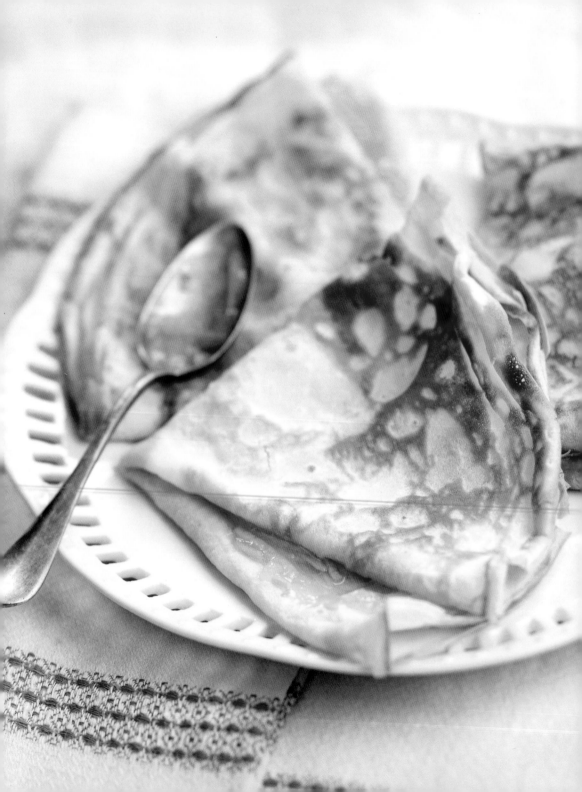

Crêpes Suzette

Crêpes are a great French culinary tradition. Classic crêpes Suzette are garnished with "beurre Suzette"—a mixture of orange juice and zest, sugar, softened butter, and Grand Marnier or Cointreau. Here, the batter is made lighter with the use of cornstarch (cornflour) and fat-free milk. The classic taste is preserved by flambéing the crêpes with liqueur before filling them with an orange sauce.

PREP TIME 20 minutes | **REST TIME** 20 minutes | **CHILL TIME** 20 minutes |
COOK TIME 15 minutes

INGREDIENTS FOR 4 PEOPLE
Scant ½ cup (2 oz./60 g) all-purpose
   (plain) flour
⅓ cup (2 oz./60 g) cornstarch (cornflour)
2 tablespoons powdered sweetener
   for cooking
Pinch of salt
2 eggs
1 ¼ cups (10 fl. oz./300 ml) fat-free milk
1 teaspoon sunflower oil

FOR THE FILLING
2 untreated oranges
3 tablespoons (1 oz./25 g) cornstarch
   (cornflour)
2 tablespoons powdered sweetener
   for cooking
4 teaspoons orange-flavored liqueur
   (e.g. Cointreau or Grand Marnier)

1   Make the crêpe batter. In a bowl, sift together the flour, cornstarch, and sweetener. Add a pinch of salt and the eggs. Mix well until smooth. Gradually pour in the fat-free milk, whisking constantly to prevent the batter becoming lumpy. Let the batter stand for 20 minutes.

2   Make 4 thin crêpes in a lightly oiled nonstick pancake pan.

3   Wash the oranges and zest them. Cut the oranges in half and juice. In a small saucepan, mix the orange juice and zest, the cornstarch, and the sweetener. Cook, stirring, over a low heat until the mixture thickens. Cool, then refrigerate for 20 minutes.

4   Heat the pancake pan. Fold each crêpe in quarters (like a fan), place in the pan, pour over the orange liqueur, and flambé. To serve, remove the crêpes from the pan, open in half, place on individual plates, and pour over the orange sauce.

Mini chocolate-chip brioches
Mini-brioches aux pépites de chocolat

Brioches are viennoiseries made from yeast-leavened dough that is rich in eggs, flour, and butter. You can find them braided in the Vendée region, flavored with orange flower water in the southeast of France, and garnished with sugar-coated almonds in Savoie. So that you can enjoy them too, this recipe uses fat-free milk, light butter, and sweetener and contains only half the amount of fat and sugar as traditional recipes.

PREP TIME 25 minutes | **REST TIME** 20 minutes | **COOK TIME** 20 minutes

INGREDIENTS FOR 4 PEOPLE
⅓ oz. (8 g) fresh baker's yeast
1 egg
Scant ¼ cup (1 ¾ fl. oz./50 ml) fat-free milk
2 tablespoons powdered sweetener for cooking
Generous ½ cup (2 oz./60 g) cake (soft white) flour
⅓ cup (2 oz./60 g) cornstarch (cornflour)
3 tablespoons (1 ½ oz./45 g) light butter, softened
¼ cup (1 ½ oz./40 g) dark (unsweetened) chocolate chips
A little oil for greasing the molds

1 Dissolve the yeast in a little warm water. In a bowl, mix the egg, milk, and sweetener. Add the dissolved yeast and sift in the flour and cornstarch. Fold in. Knead the dough vigorously until it becomes elastic, smooth, and no longer sticks to your fingers. Incorporate the softened butter, then the chocolate chips.

2 Lightly oil four small molds. Divide the dough between the molds so it fills them to about one third full. Fill a large saucepan with hot water, cover with a heat-resistant plate, place the brioche molds on top, and cover with a clean dish cloth (tea towel). Let rise for 20 minutes. The dough should double in volume.

3 Meanwhile, preheat the oven to 425°F (220°C/Gas mark 8). Bake the brioches in the oven for 15–20 minutes (the time will vary depending on the thickness of the dough). Avoid opening the oven door for the first 10 minutes of cooking time.

4 Turn out the brioches and let cool before eating. You can vary the flavors and garnishes: try adding orange flower water, vanilla extract, or 1 oz. (30 g) of mixed dried fruit.

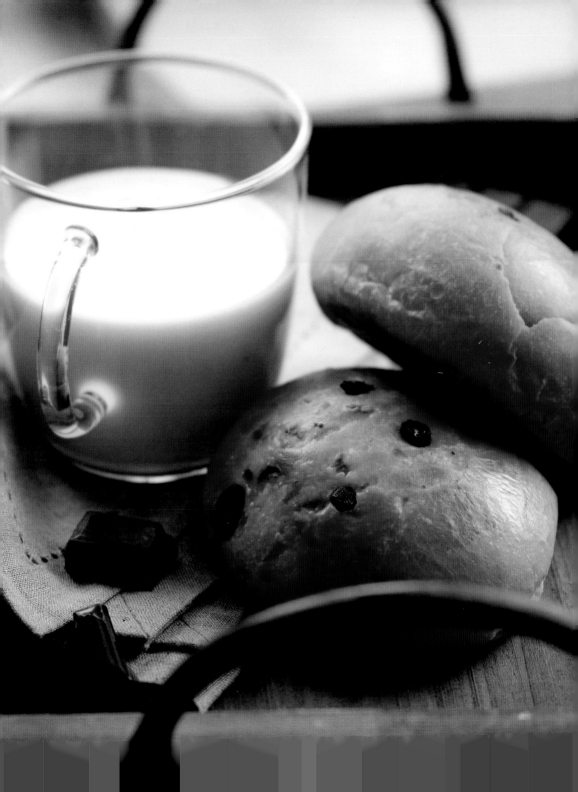

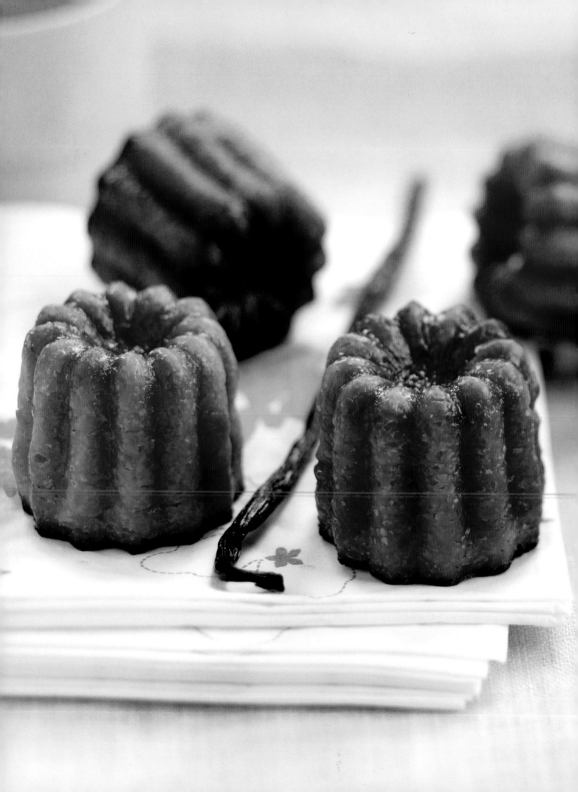

Cannelés

Specialties of Bordeaux, cannelés are little cakes with melt-in-the-mouth centers and a thick, caramelized crust. Using sweetener and cornstarch (cornflour) enables you to enjoy a lighter version, with the delicious taste of vanilla and rum.

PREP TIME 15 minutes | **CHILL TIME** 24 hours | **COOK TIME** 1 hour 25 minutes

INGREDIENTS FOR 4 PEOPLE
1 vanilla bean (pod)
2 cups (1 pint/500 ml) reduced-fat (semi-skimmed) milk
½ cup (2 oz./60 g) cake (soft white) flour
⅓ cup (2 oz./60 g) cornstarch (cornflour)
6 tablespoons powdered sweetener for cooking
Pinch of salt
2 whole eggs + 2 egg yolks
¼ cup (1 ¾ oz./50 g) superfine (caster) sugar
2 tablespoons rum

1   Slit the vanilla bean in two and heat in a small saucepan with the milk. Remove from the heat as soon as the milk begins to simmer and let infuse.

2   Meanwhile, sift the flour and cornstarch into a bowl and stir in the sweetener and salt. Make a well in the center and add the eggs and egg yolks, sugar, and rum. Mix well.

3   Remove the vanilla bean from the milk, pour the warm milk over the mixture in the bowl, and stir in well. Let cool and cover the bowl with plastic wrap. Refrigerate for 24 hours.

4   Preheat the oven to 300°F (150°C/Gas mark 2). Fill silicone *cannelé* or mini-muffin molds three quarters full with the mixture and bake in the oven for 1 ¼ hours.

5   Serve the *cannelés* warm or cold.

Jelly (Swiss) roll
Biscuit roulé allégé

This dessert has simple ingredients but requires a certain amount of skill to make. As it is made from cornstarch (cornflour) and other light ingredients, you no longer need to turn down this favorite among the young and old alike!

PREP TIME 30 minutes | **COOK TIME** 10 minutes

INGREDIENTS FOR 4 PEOPLE
4 eggs
Pinch of salt
¼ cup (1 ¾ oz./50 g) superfine (caster) sugar
4 tablespoons powdered sweetener for cooking
1 tablespoon baking powder
5 tablespoons (1 ¾ oz./50 g) cornstarch (cornflour)
Generous ⅓ cup (1 ¾ oz./50 g) all-purpose (plain) flour
2 teaspoons (⅓ oz./10 g) light butter
⅓ cup (3 ½ oz./100 g) jelly (jam) of your choice
4 tablespoons light unsweetened cocoa powder (for decoration)

1   Preheat the oven to 400°F (200°C/Gas mark 6).

2   Separate the egg whites from the yolks. Whisk the egg whites until firm with a pinch of salt. In a separate, large bowl, whisk the egg yolks, sugar, and sweetener until the mixture turns pale. Sift in the baking powder, cornstarch, and flour and mix well. Carefully fold in the whisked egg whites.

3   Line a baking tray (or jelly/Swiss roll pan) with lightly buttered parchment (greaseproof) paper. Pour the cake batter into the tray, spreading it evenly over the surface. Bake in the oven for about 10 minutes. The cake is ready when it is pulling away from the edges.

4   As soon as you remove it from the oven, turn it out carefully onto a clean damp dish cloth (tea towel) and roll it up so that it takes its shape. Unroll, spread the jelly over the whole surface, and roll up again. Trim the ends of the cake and dust with cocoa powder before serving. To make mini-rolls, roll the sponge lengthwise, follow the instructions above, then cut into individual portions.

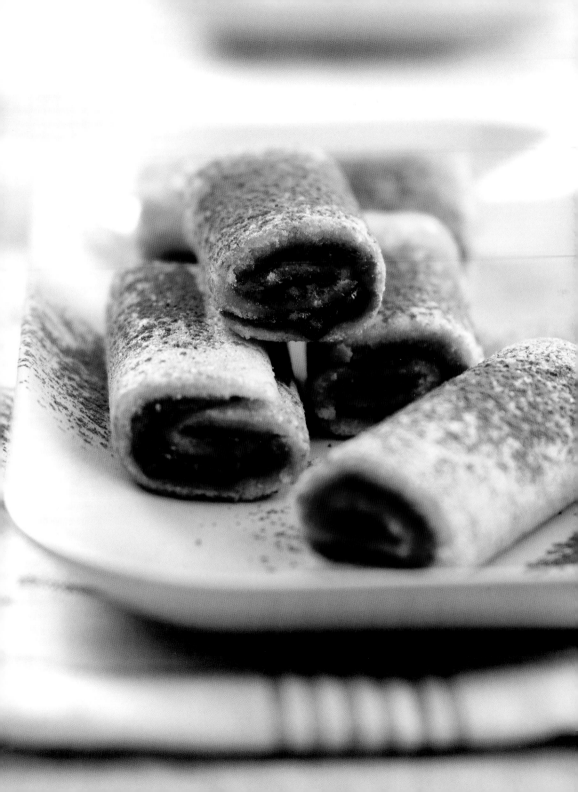

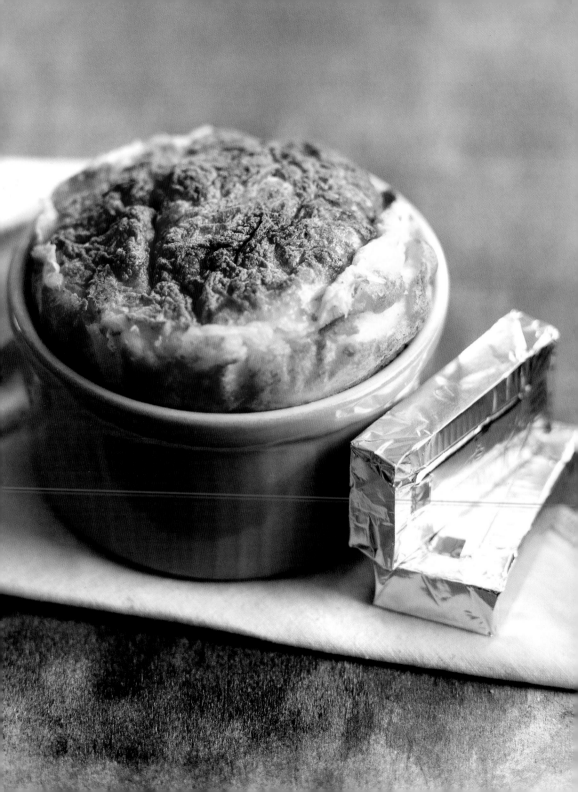

Individual cheese soufflés
Petits soufflés légers au fromage

A healthy butter-free white sauce made with fat-free milk, just the right amount of cheese, half-and-half (single cream), and a single egg yolk—so you need no longer resist classic cheese soufflé on the basis that it's too high in fat!

PREP TIME 25 minutes | **COOK TIME** 30 minutes

INGREDIENTS FOR 4 PEOPLE
2 tablespoons cornstarch (cornflour)
⅔ cup (5 ½ fl oz./160 ml) half-and-half (single cream)
Scant ¼ cup (1 ¾ fl oz./50 ml) fat-free milk
2 light creamy Swiss cheese wedges
1 egg + 3 egg whites
¾ cup (3 ½ oz./100 g) grated Swiss cheese
½ teaspoon grated nutmeg
Salt and pepper

1   Preheat the oven to 400°F (200°C/Gas mark 6).

2   Line four individual ramekins with parchment (greaseproof) paper or use individual silicone molds.

3   Dissolve the cornstarch in the half-and-half and milk. Bring to a boil, stirring continuously, until the mixture thickens. Remove from the heat, add the light Swiss cheese wedges, stir to mix in well, and let cool.

4   Separate the egg whites from the yolks. Add the egg yolk to the sauce mixture, then stir in the grated Swiss cheese, nutmeg, and salt and pepper. Mix well.

5   Whisk the egg whites with a pinch of salt until stiff and add them to the sauce. Fold in carefully to retain the air. Pour the mixture into the ramekins and bake in the oven for 20 minutes without opening the oven door during cooking.

6   The soufflés are ready when they have risen well and turned golden brown. Serve immediately.

Leek and Maroilles cheese tart
Tarte fine poireaux-maroilles

A specialty of northern France, flamiche is made with puff pastry (known for its high butter content) and a large quantity of the famous local cheese Maroilles. Our recipe, which combines softened and browned leeks with Maroilles cheese on a very light phyllo (filo) pastry base, will delight your tastebuds and enable you to enjoy these traditional French flavors without piling on the calories.

PREP TIME 30 minutes | **COOK TIME** 40 minutes

INGREDIENTS FOR 4 PEOPLE
14 oz. (400 g) trimmed leeks
1 onion
3 phyllo (filo) pastry sheets
1 egg
4 tablespoons low-fat sour cream (crème fraîche)
3 ½ oz. (100 g) Maroilles (or other strong-tasting soft cheese), thinly sliced
Salt and pepper

1   Preheat the oven to 350°F (180°C/Gas mark 4).

2   Wash the leeks thoroughly. Cut the white and soft green parts into thin slices and steam for 15 minutes.

3   Meanwhile, peel and finely chop the onion. Dry-fry the onion in a nonstick skillet (frying pan) until golden. Remove from the heat and stir in the cooked leeks.

4   Line a small pie plate (flan tin) with a sheet of parchment (greaseproof) paper, then with the three phyllo pastry sheets, laying them one over the other. Prebake for 10 minutes in the oven.

5   Meanwhile, in a bowl, beat together the egg and the cream. Season with salt and pepper. Cover the pastry sheets with the leek and onion mixture then pour over the beaten egg and cream. Lay the cheese slices over the top and bake in the center of the oven for 15 minutes, until the cheese has turned golden brown.

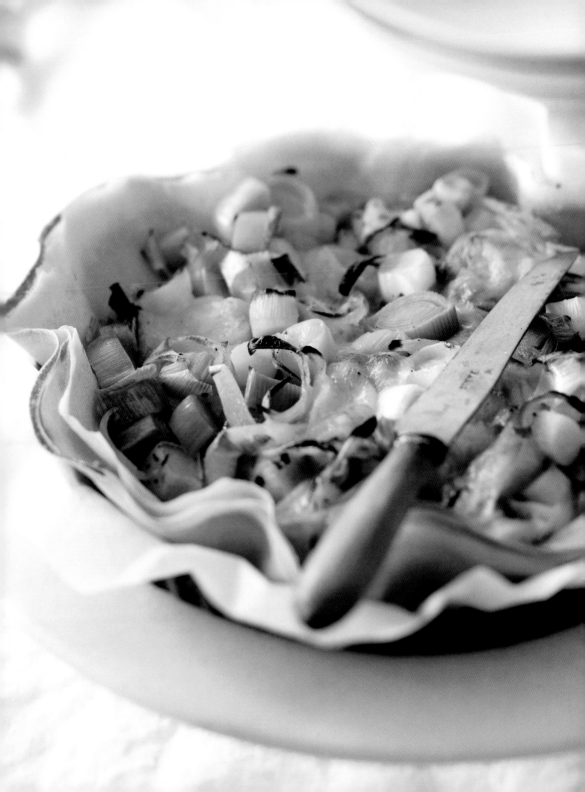

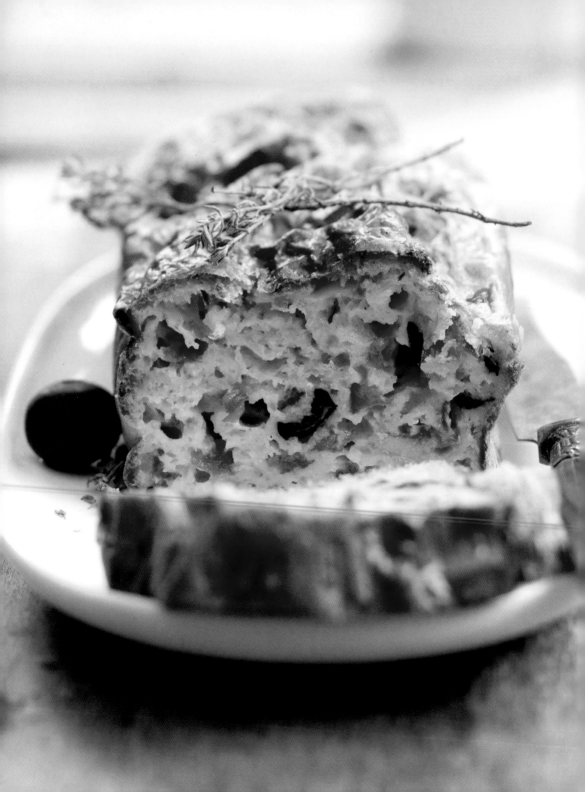

Smoked bacon, olive, and bell pepper loaf
Cake léger bacon, olives et poivrons

Savory loaf cakes, often served with aperitifs in France, are frequently criticized for being heavy to digest, especially when they contain—in addition to butter—bacon and olives! But this low-calorie version is made with a light cake batter containing plain nonfat yogurt and filled with peppers and lean smoked Canadian (back) bacon.

PREP TIME 25 minutes | **REST TIME** 15 minutes | **COOK TIME** 55 minutes

INGREDIENTS FOR 4 PEOPLE

1 small red bell pepper (3 ½ oz./100 g)
⅔ cup (3 oz./80 g) all-purpose (plain) flour
1 ½ teaspoons baking powder
1 egg
½ cup (4 ½ oz./125 g) plain nonfat yogurt
1 teaspoon olive oil

3 ½ oz. (100 g) sliced smoked Canadian-style (back) bacon (fat removed)
8 black olives
1 sprig thyme
A few fresh basil leaves
1 teaspoon ground cumin
Salt and pepper

1 Preheat the oven to 400°F (200°C/Gas mark 6).

2 Wash the pepper, cut in half, and remove the core and seeds. Cook the pepper halves in the oven for 10 minutes, cut side up. Turn them over and cook for an additional 10 minutes until the skins are well browned. Leave the oven on.

3 Put the hot peppers in a sealable plastic bag and let rest for 15 minutes. When you remove them from the bag, the skins will peel off easily.

4 Sift the flour and baking powder into a bowl. In a separate bowl, beat together the egg, yogurt, and oil using a fork. Pour over the flour and stir the mixture together with a whisk until you have a smooth batter.

5 Cut the smoked bacon into thin strips, dice the peppers, and chop the olives (pitting them first if necessary). Remove the leaves from the thyme sprig and chop the basil leaves and stir into the cake batter along with the ground cumin, bacon, peppers, olives, and salt and pepper. Pour into a prepared loaf pan.

6 Bake in the oven for 35 minutes. Let cool then remove from the pan, cut into slices, and serve with salad.

Zucchini flower fritters
Beignets de fleurs de courgette

Fritters are usually high in fat because they're deep-fried in oil. Discover this largely forgotten—yet deliciously crunchy—recipe in a light version, in which the fritters are oven-baked rather than deep-fried.

PREP TIME 15 minutes | **COOK TIME** 15 minutes

INGREDIENTS FOR 4 PEOPLE
24 zucchini (courgette) flowers
1 egg
¾ cup (3 oz./80 g) cornstarch (cornflour)
1 teaspoon olive oil
⅔ cup (5 fl oz./150 ml) fat-free milk
1 bunch parsley
Salt and pepper

1 Clean the zucchini flowers and remove the stems and the pistils in their centers. Place them flower-side down on a dish and set aside.

2 Preheat the oven to 350°F (180°C/Gas mark 4).

3 Separate the egg white and yolk. Sift the cornstarch into a bowl, make a well in the center, and add the egg yolk, a pinch of salt, and the olive oil. Using a whisk, mix the ingredients together well then add the milk a little at a time, continuing to whisk.

4 In a separate bowl, beat the egg white with a pinch of salt using a whisk until it forms peaks, and fold it into the batter. Chop the parsley and stir into the batter with salt and pepper.

5 Cover a large baking sheet with parchment (greaseproof) paper. Dip the zucchini flowers into the batter then place them on the baking sheet. Cook in the oven for 15 minutes. Serve the fritters while they're still warm.

Crispy seafood cups
on a bed of baby salad leaves

*Timbales croquantes aux fruits de mer
sur lit de jeunes pousses*

Made with puff pastry and white sauce, traditional vol-au-vents are rich in butter. These crispy cups made with phyllo (filo) pastry look lovely and their light seafood filling will delight your dinner guests.

PREP TIME 40 minutes | **COOK TIME** 1 hour

INGREDIENTS FOR 4 PEOPLE

4 phyllo (filo) pastry sheets	1 lb. (500 g) frozen mixed seafood
2 shallots	¼ cup (1 oz./25 g) cornstarch (cornflour)
14 oz. (400 g) mushrooms	Scant 1 cup (7 fl oz./200 ml) fat-free milk
1 sprig tarragon	½ teaspoon grated nutmeg
2 teaspoons vegetable bouillon powder	14 oz. (400 g) mixed baby salad leaves
	Salt and pepper

1 Preheat the oven to 350°F (180°C/Gas mark 4). Upturn four small ovenproof bowls on a baking sheet and cover with strips of phyllo pastry. Bake in the oven until golden and crispy. Remove from the oven and let cool on the bowls.

2 Peel and finely chop the shallots. Dry-fry in a nonstick sauté pan until translucent. Wipe the mushrooms with damp paper towels and remove and discard the mushroom stalks. Finely chop the mushrooms. Add them to the shallots and cook for 15 minutes, stirring. Stir in the snipped tarragon and set aside.

3 In a large pan, dissolve the vegetable bouillon powder in a scant cup (7 fl oz./200 ml) of water and bring to a boil. Reduce the heat, tip the seafood into the stock, and simmer for 10 minutes. Drain the seafood, reserving the cooking liquid. In a saucepan, dissolve the cornstarch in the cold milk, then mix into the reserved cooking liquid. Add the nutmeg, salt, and pepper and heat, stirring, until the mixture thickens. Tip in the drained seafood and the mushrooms, mix in well and heat for 5 minutes, stirring.

4 Divide the salad leaves between four plates, place a phyllo pastry shell on top and carefully fill with the seafood mixture. Serve immediately.

Smoked salmon on buckwheat blinis with sour cream sauce

Saumon fumé, blinis légers au sarrasin et sauce fraîche

Smoked salmon is often served with blinis and sour cream (or crème fraîche) on special occasions. Although it's perfectly acceptable to eat smoked salmon on a weight-loss diet, blinis and cream need to be limited, but this recipe will allow you to enjoy this combination of foods while still reducing your calorie intake thanks to the light batter used to make the blinis and a sauce made from nonfat fromage blanc or yogurt.

PREP TIME 20 minutes | **REST TIME** 30 minutes | **COOK TIME** 40 minutes

INGREDIENTS FOR 4 PEOPLE
1 ½ cups (14 oz./400 g) nonfat fromage blanc or plain nonfat regular or Greek yogurt
½ lemon
8 fresh chives
4 slices smoked salmon
Salt and pepper

FOR THE 12 BLINIS
½ cup (2 ¼ oz./65 g) buckwheat flour
⅔ cup (2 ¼ oz./65 g) cornstarch (cornflour)
2 teaspoons (10 g) baking powder
2 eggs
⅓ cup (2.75 fl oz./80 ml) low-fat sour cream (crème fraîche)
Scant 1 cup (7 fl oz./200 ml) fat-free milk
Pinch of salt

1 To make the blinis, in a bowl, mix together the buckwheat flour, cornstarch, baking powder, and salt. Make a well in the center. Break the eggs into this well and mix them gently into the dry ingredients until you have a smooth batter, then add the cream. Add the milk a little at a time. The batter should be completely smooth. Cover the bowl with a clean dish cloth (tea towel) and let rest for 30 minutes at room temperature.

2 Meanwhile, mix together the fromage blanc or yogurt with the lemon juice, snipped chives (reserving some for decoration), salt and pepper. Set aside in the refrigerator.

3 Heat a small nonstick pan. (If necessary to prevent sticking, you can wipe the surface with a lightly oiled piece of absorbent paper towels.) Drop a tablespoonful of batter in the pan and cook for 1–1 ½ minutes on each side. Continue to make 12 blinis.

4 To serve, place three blinis on each plate. Put a spoonful of sauce on top, then lay a slice of smoked salmon in the center and decorate with the reserved snipped chives.

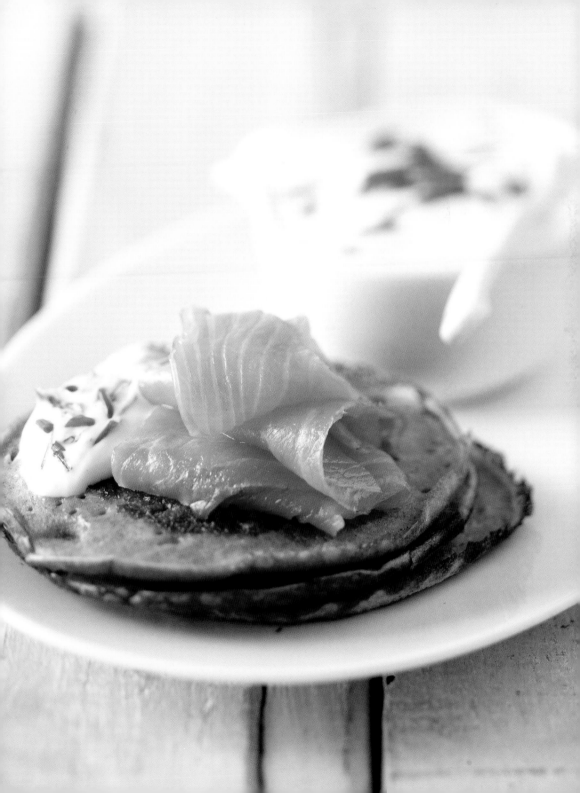

Onion soup au gratin
Soupe à l'oignon gratinée des Halles

It's easy to double the number of calories in this favorite of French gastronomy if you're too liberal with the cheese. Here's how to enjoy this delicious dish by making it with a limited quantity of fat and a reasonable amount of bread and toasted cheese. No more reason to resist temptation!

PREP TIME 20 minutes | **COOK TIME** 40 minutes

INGREDIENTS FOR 4 PEOPLE
1 medium (7 oz./200 g) onion
1 teaspoon sunflower oil
6 cups (3 pints/1.5 liters) chicken stock
⅔ cup (5 fl oz./150 ml) dry white wine
8 slices (4 ½ oz./125 g) baguette (French stick),
    toasted
⅔ cup (3 oz./80 g) grated Swiss cheese
Pepper

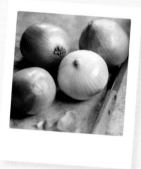

1   Peel and finely chop the onion. Heat a large nonstick cooking pot with the teaspoon of oil and sauté the chopped onion for 8 minutes over a medium heat, stirring regularly to prevent it burning. When the onion is soft and lightly browned, pour in the chicken stock and white wine, stir well, add pepper to taste, and simmer for 20 minutes.

2   Heat the oven broiler (grill) to its highest temperature. Lay half the toasted bread slices in the bottom of a soufflé dish and cover with half the grated cheese. Pour the onion soup over the top, being careful not to fill the dish to more than half full. Arrange the remaining toast slices on top and sprinkle with the remaining grated cheese. Place in the oven to brown the top for 10–15 minutes. Note: the browning must be done quickly so that the bread doesn't have time to disintegrate into the soup.

3   Serve hot.

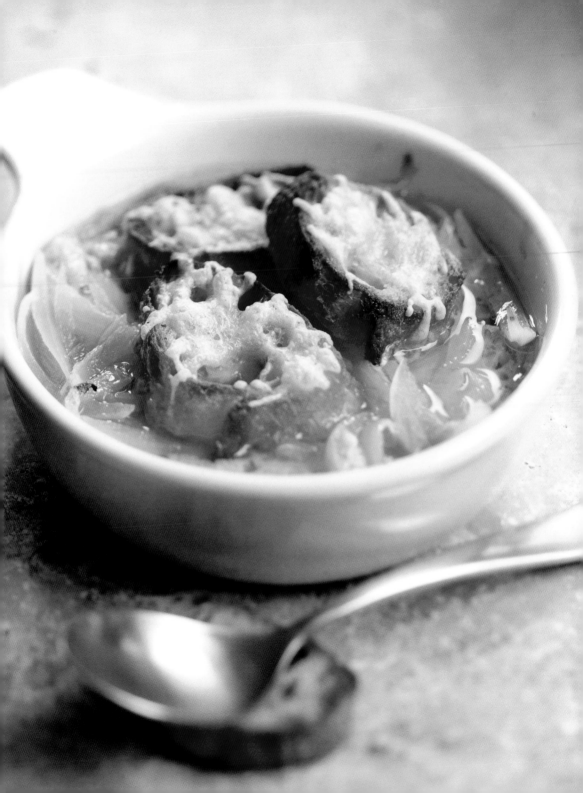

Burgundy-style poached eggs
Œufs en meurette

Discover this classic Burgundy dish made with eggs but also containing butter, wine, and often bacon, revisited here in a light version—notably in fats—that will fit perfectly into a weight-loss diet.

PREP TIME 35 minutes | **COOK TIME** 35 minutes

INGREDIENTS FOR 4 PEOPLE

2 onions
2 carrots
1 leek, white parts only
4 cloves garlic
2 cups (1 pint/500 ml) red Burgundy wine
1 bouquet garni
½ teaspoon sugar
1 tablespoon (½ oz./15 g) light butter, softened
1 tablespoon (⅓ oz./10 g) cornstarch (cornflour)
1 tablespoon white alcohol vinegar
4 very fresh eggs
4 slices (2 ¼ oz./60 g) baguette (French stick)
1 tablespoon snipped chives
Salt and pepper

1 Peel and finely chop the onions. Peel the carrots, wash them, and chop them into small dice. Wash and slice the leek. Peel and crush the garlic.

2 Pour the wine into a large pan and add the onions, carrots, leek, garlic, bouquet garni, sugar, and a little salt and pepper. Bring to a boil, reduce the heat, and simmer without covering for 15 minutes.

3 Strain, then return the wine to the pan and reduce until you have about 2–2 ½ cups (1–1 ½ pints/ 500–600 ml). It should have a slightly syrupy consistency. Flambé to evaporate the alcohol.

4 Mix together the softened butter and the cornstarch to make a beurre manié. Add this mixture to the wine a little at a time, stirring constantly, until the sauce simmers and thickens. Let simmer gently for 2 minutes then check the seasoning: add more salt and pepper if needed.

5 Meanwhile, half fill a sauté pan with water and bring to a boil. Add the vinegar and simmer. Break an egg into a cup and tip it quickly into the pan where the water is boiling the most vigorously. Spoon the white over the yolk using a slotted spoon. Repeat with the remaining eggs and reduce the heat so that the water is simmering gently. Let the eggs poach for 3 minutes, then check that they're cooked by lifting out an egg using a slotted spoon: the white should have solidified but the egg should still feel soft in the center for a creamy yolk. Keep the poached eggs warm in another pan of warm water.

6 Toast the French bread slices under the broiler (grill) or in a toaster.

7 Drain the poached eggs on a clean dish cloth (tea towel) and, using a knife, cut away any stray bits of egg white so that the eggs are regularly shaped.

8 Put a slice of toasted French bread in each of four shallow dishes, place a poached egg on top, and pour over the wine sauce. Garnish with a few snipped chives and serve immediately.

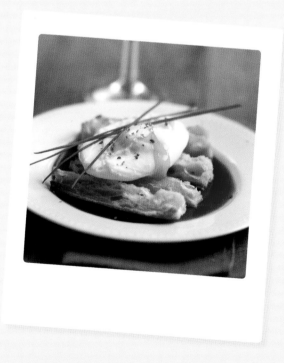

Pissaladière niçoise

You might think you'd need to banish this delicious Mediterranean specialty from the menu, but in fact, the calorie count of this dish depends mainly on the amount of olive oil you use. As 2 teaspoons of oil contain 90 kcal, you'll understand that adding more can cause the calorific value of the dish to rise rapidly! With this light recipe and carefully measured ingredients, you can enjoy it guilt-free.

PREP TIME 35 minutes | **REST TIME** 2 hours 15 minutes | **COOK TIME** 45 minutes

INGREDIENTS FOR 4 PEOPLE
4 medium (1 lb./500 g) onions
1 teaspoon olive oil
1 teaspoon herbes de Provence
12 anchovy fillets (not in oil), desalted
4 black olives
Salt and pepper

FOR THE PIZZA DOUGH
½ tablespoon (¼ oz./8 g) active dry yeast
Scant ½ cup (3 ½ fl oz./100 ml)
 + 2 tablespoons warm water
1 ½ cups (7 oz./200 g) all-purpose (plain) flour
1 teaspoon salt

1 Make the pizza dough. Dissolve the yeast in the 2 tablespoons of warm water (95°F/35°C), then add the scant ½ cup (3 ½ fl oz./100 ml) warm water. Let rest for 15 minutes.

2 Sift the flour and salt into a mixing bowl and make a well in the center. Pour the yeast mixture into the center and mix in the flour a little at a time. Knead until the dough is smooth and elastic. Form into a ball. Cover the bowl with a clean, damp dish cloth (tea towel) and let rest for 2 hours in a warm, draft-free place.

3 Knead the dough again and divide into four equal-size pieces. Stretch each piece into a pancake shape and lightly roll the edges to make a rim. Prick the center of each pizza base using a fork. Preheat the oven to 350°F (180°C/Gas mark 4).

4 Peel and finely chop the onions. Heat the olive oil in a nonstick sauté pan and fry the onions for 10 minutes to soften but not brown them. Add a little salt, pepper, and sprinkle with the herbes de Provence. Stir in and remove the pan from the heat.

5 Place the pizza bases on a baking sheet and cover with some of the onions. Arrange 3 anchovy fillets and a whole black olive on each one. Place in the oven and bake for about 30 minutes. Serve immediately.

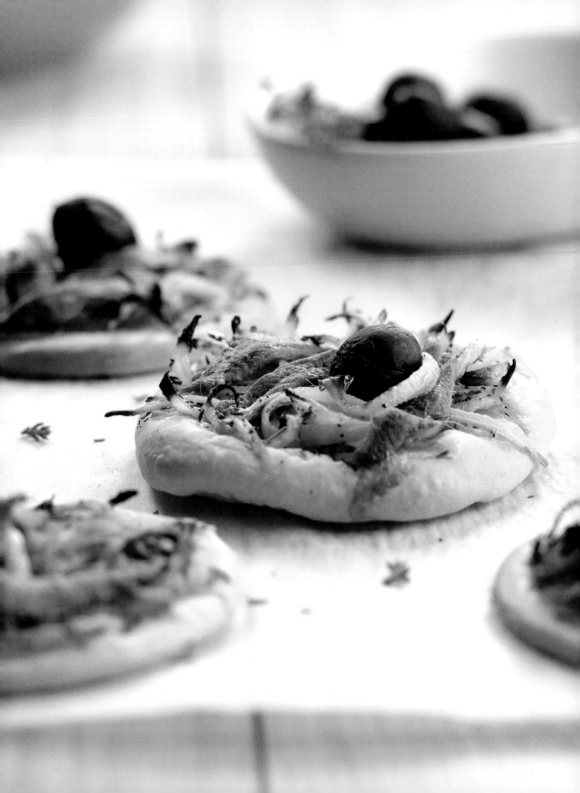

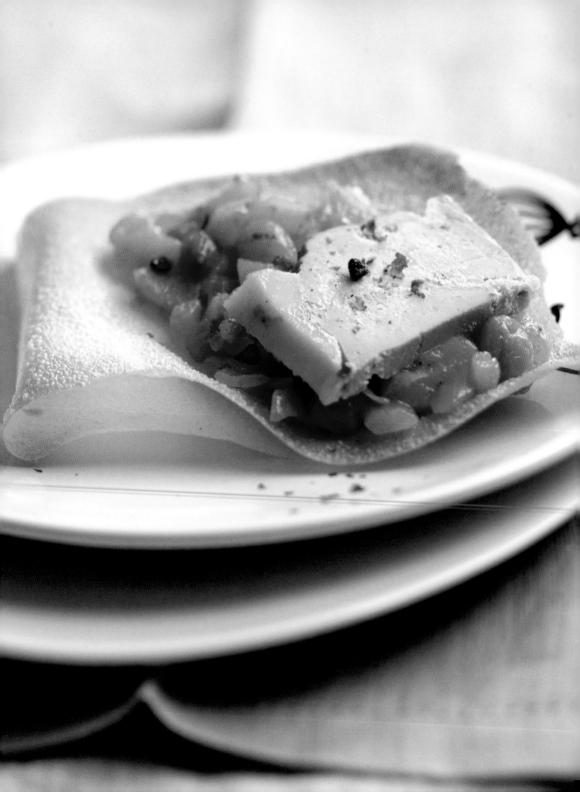

Foie gras tartlets with apple chutney

Tartelettes de foie gras au chutney de pommes

No French celebration is complete without foie gras on the dinner menu. Served very simply in slices to preserve its subtle flavors, it is usually accompanied by toasted brioche and a spoonful of various vegetable- or fruit-based chutneys. Here the proportions are revisited, with a simple phyllo (filo) pastry tartlet to provide crispiness and a good dollop of apple chutney naturally sweetened with raisins to bring out the flavor of the foie gras.

PREP TIME 20 minutes | **COOK TIME** 1 hour 15 minutes

INGREDIENTS FOR 4 PEOPLE

2 onions
4 apples, preferably Golden Delicious
3 tablespoons (1oz./30 g) raisins
½ teaspoon ground ginger
½ teaspoon curry powder
4 teaspoons powdered sweetener for cooking

Scant ½ cup (3 ½ fl oz./100 ml) cider vinegar
2 phyllo (filo) pastry sheets
5 ½ oz. (160 g) whole foie gras, cut into 4 slices
Salt and freshly ground pepper

1 Peel and finely chop the onions and dry-fry them gently in a nonstick saucepan. Wash, peel, and core the apples and cut them into small pieces. When the onions have lightly browned, add the apple and cook for a few minutes. Reduce the heat and add the raisins, spices, sweetener, and a pinch of salt. Stir together and add the vinegar. Cover the pan and cook over a low heat for 1 hour, checking the pan and adding a little water as necessary to prevent the chutney drying out or sticking to the pan. Let cool.

2 Heat the broiler (grill). Cut the phyllo pastry sheets in half and fold them so that they're the right size to hold a slice of foie gras. Place under the broiler until lightly golden on each side, then let cool.

3 To serve, place a phyllo pastry base on each of four side plates, spoon the apple chutney on top, and finish with a slice of foie gras. Grind some pepper on top and serve immediately.

Salade lyonnaise

This Lyon specialty is not particularly high in fat but when you're following a weight-loss program it's good to find ways of reducing the calorie content of each dish. Here, smoked streaky bacon has been replaced with Canadian (back) bacon, which is equally rich in flavor but much lower in fat content. Croutons, which are real oil sponges, have been swapped for simple cubes of toasted bread.

PREP TIME 20 minutes | **COOK TIME** 10 minutes

INGREDIENTS FOR 4 PEOPLE
14 oz. (400 g) dandelion leaves
2 tablespoons white alcohol vinegar
7 oz. (200 g) lean smoked Canadian-
   style (back) bacon
4 slices (2 oz./60 g) wholegrain bread
4 eggs
Fresh chives

FOR THE DRESSING
4 teaspoons canola (rapeseed) oil
2 teaspoons vinegar
1 teaspoon traditional wholegrain mustard
Salt and pepper

1 Sort and wash well the dandelion leaves in water to which 1 tablespoon of the vinegar has been added.

2 Cut the smoked bacon into thin strips. Toast the bread and cut it into cubes. Brown the bacon in a nonstick, pan then dry-fry the toast cubes in the same pan. Meanwhile, poach the eggs: bring a pan of water to a boil and add the remaining tablespoon of vinegar. Break an egg into a cup, then tip it into the water; using a cup will prevent the egg white from dispersing. After 1–1 ½ minutes, the egg will be "soft-poached": remove it carefully from the pan using a slotted spoon and drain it in a bowl. Repeat to poach the remaining eggs.

3 Make the dressing: shake all the ingredients together in a screw-top jar until combined. Divide the dandelion leaves seasoned with the dressing between four plates. Sprinkle the hot bacon and croutons over, top each plate with a still-warm poached egg, and garnish with snipped chives. Serve immediately.

Cheese puffs
Gougères

For a low-calorie hors d'oeuvre, let yourself be tempted by these small light cheese puffs. Here, the quantities of the ingredients have simply been adapted to make a lighter version of gougères that are quick to make and can be enjoyed with a clear conscience.

PREP TIME 25 minutes | **COOK TIME** 25 minutes

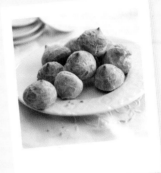

INGREDIENTS FOR 4 PEOPLE
1 tablespoon (½ oz./15 g) cake (soft white) flour
1 ½ tablespoons (½ oz./15 g) cornstarch (cornflour)
1 ½ tablespoons (¾ oz./20 g) light butter
4 tablespoons water
Pinch of salt
1 egg
1 ¼ cups (5 oz./150 g) grated light Swiss cheese

1 Preheat the oven to 425°F (220°C/Gas mark 8).

2 Sift the flour and cornstarch into a bowl. Cut the butter into pieces and put into a saucepan with the water and a pinch of salt. Bring to a boil. As soon as it begins to boil, remove the pan from the heat, tip in the sifted flour and cornstarch and mix vigorously using a wooden spoon. The mixture will swell and form a ball that will separate from the pan. If this doesn't happen spontaneously, put the pan back over a low heat and stir until the dough is sufficiently dry to unstick from the pan.

3 Beat the egg. Remove the pan from the heat and mix in the egg. Check the consistency of the dough: it should be sufficiently firm and supple. Add the grated cheese and incorporate well.

4 Cover a baking sheet with parchment (greaseproof) paper. Divide the choux pastry into small lumps (about 10 or so). Bake in the center of the oven for 15–20 minutes until the *gougères* are risen and golden.

Tomato tart
Tarte à la tomate

A French version of pizza, this tomato tart is to die for! You won't have to deprive yourself if you adopt this healthy recipe that uses special puff pastry made from nonfat petits-suisses (French cream cheese from Normandy; if unavailable, substitute fat-free cottage cheese and nonfat Greek yogurt)—a real calorie-saver for a traditional pleasure!

PREP TIME 20 minutes | **REST TIME** 30 minutes | **COOK TIME** 55 minutes

INGREDIENTS FOR 4 PEOPLE
4 tomatoes
4 tablespoons strong prepared
   mustard
1 teaspoon herbes de Provence
Salt and pepper

FOR THE PUFF PASTRY
Scant ½ cup (2 ¾ oz./75 g) all-purpose (plain)
   flour + a little for dusting the work surface
Scant ½ cup (2 ¾ oz./75 g) cornstarch
   (cornflour)
Pinch of sugar
1 stick (4 oz./120 g) light butter, chilled
4 plain nonfat petits-suisses, or 6 tablespoons
   (30 oz./85g) fat-free cottage cheese + scant
   ½ cup (4 oz./115 g) plain nonfat Greek yogurt

1 Sift the flour and cornstarch into a bowl and stir in the sugar. Make a well in the center. Cut the chilled butter into small pieces. Drain the petits-suisses (or cottage cheese) well. Add the butter and petits-suisses (or cottage cheese and Greek yogurt) to the dry ingredients. Mix the ingredients together using your fingertips until it resembles bread crumbs. Form into a ball and, still in the bowl, cover with a clean dish cloth (tea towel). Let rest for at least 30 minutes.

2 Meanwhile, preheat the oven to 450°F (230°C/Gas mark 8).

3 Sprinkle the pastry dough and the work surface with a little flour then roll out using a rolling pin. This dough contains more water than ordinary puff pastry. Lay the pastry into the prepared pie plate (flan tin) and bake it blind for 10–15 minutes.

4 Slice the tomatoes. Spread a good quantity of mustard (more or less depending on your taste) then cover with tomato slices. Sprinkle with salt, pepper, and herbes de Provence. Bake in the oven for 40 minutes, covering with a sheet of aluminum foil halfway through the cooking time.

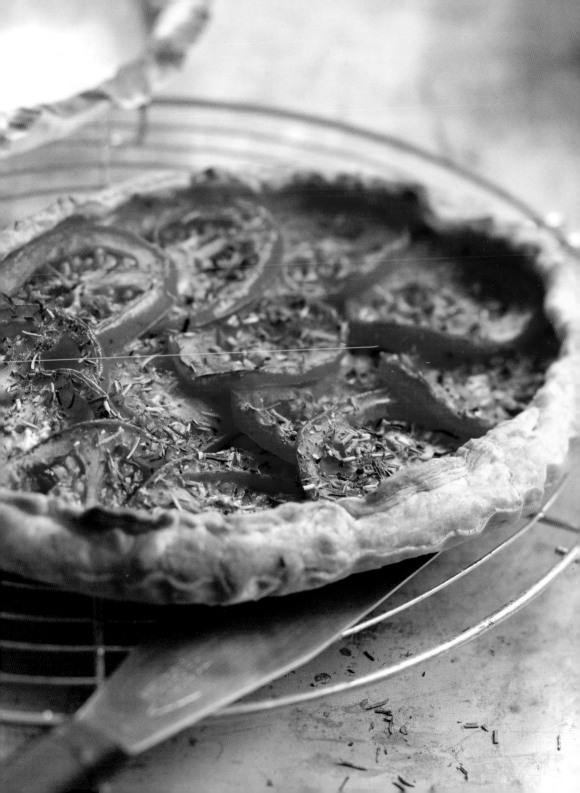

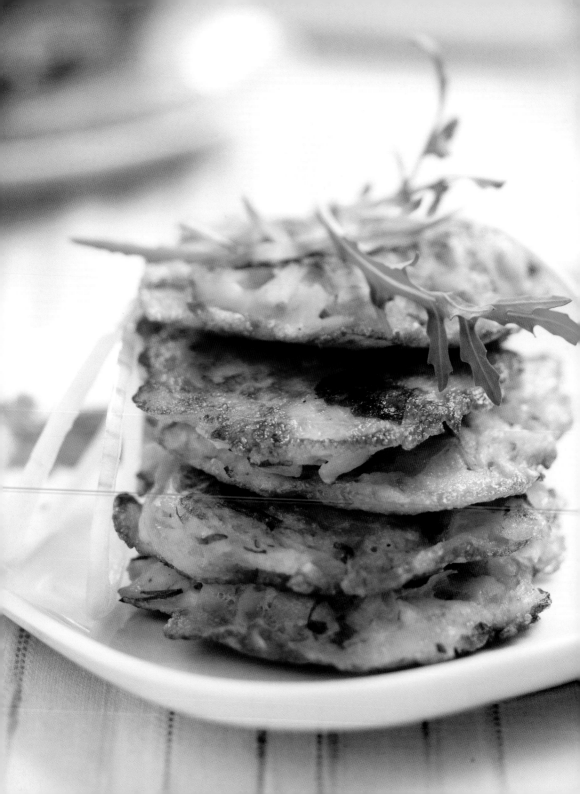

Crispy potato cakes
Croustilles de pommes de terre

The potato, the most widely consumed root vegetable, is a moderately energy-providing carbohydrate, with 24 kcal per 1 oz. (85 kcal per 100 g), but the means of cooking it can easily increase the calorie count. Here, potatoes cooked in the form of patties have a lovely crispiness with a minimum of fat.

PREP TIME 20 minutes | **COOK TIME** 15 minutes

INGREDIENTS FOR 4 PEOPLE
14 oz. (400 g) potatoes
1 onion
4 eggs
1 small bunch parsley
4 teaspoons cornstarch (cornflour)
4 teaspoons olive oil
Salt and pepper

1 Wash and peel the potatoes and grate them using the coarse grater of a food processor. Dry well. Peel and finely chop the onion. Beat the eggs and wash, dry, and chop the parsley.

2 In a mixing bowl, mix the grated potato, onion, eggs, cornstarch, salt, pepper, and chopped parsley. Form the mixture into 8 small patties and place on a plate.

3 Heat the oil in a nonstick skillet (frying pan) and fry the small patties on each side until they are golden (10–15 minutes).

4 Serve hot.

Cassoulet

A regional specialty of the Languedoc, cassoulet originated in Castelnaudary, but in fact every town has its own recipe, the only ingredient common to all of them being the white (haricot) bean. This version uses lean meat (duck fillet/breast) rather than confit of duck, chicken rather than pork sausages, vegetables in the form of tomatoes and carrots, and a limited amount of fat, preferably vegetable oil rather than the traditional goose fat, which is rich in saturated fatty acids.

PREP TIME 25 minutes | **COOK TIME** 40 minutes

INGREDIENTS FOR 4 PEOPLE
1 medium (3 ½ oz./100 g) carrot
14 oz. (400 g) duck fillets (breast)
1 onion
2 cloves garlic
4 chicken sausages
1 teaspoon olive oil
15 oz. (410 g) can white (haricot) beans
1 small can crushed (chopped) tomatoes
2 teaspoons tomato paste (purée)
1 sprig thyme
Salt and pepper

1 Wash and peel the carrot. Cut into slices and steam for 15 minutes. Cut the duck into thin strips and peel and chop the onion. Peel and crush the garlic.

2 Dry-fry the sausages in a large nonstick sauté pan. Set aside on a plate. In the same pan, heat the teaspoon of oil and sauté the onion, then add the duck fillet strips and cook until golden. Add the beans, crushed tomatoes, carrots, crushed garlic, salt, and pepper, and stir to mix. Lay the sausages on top.

3 Dilute the tomato paste in 1 cup (½ pint/250 ml) of water and pour into the pan. Add the thyme sprig and simmer for 20 minutes. Add more water during cooking if necessary.

4 Serve hot.

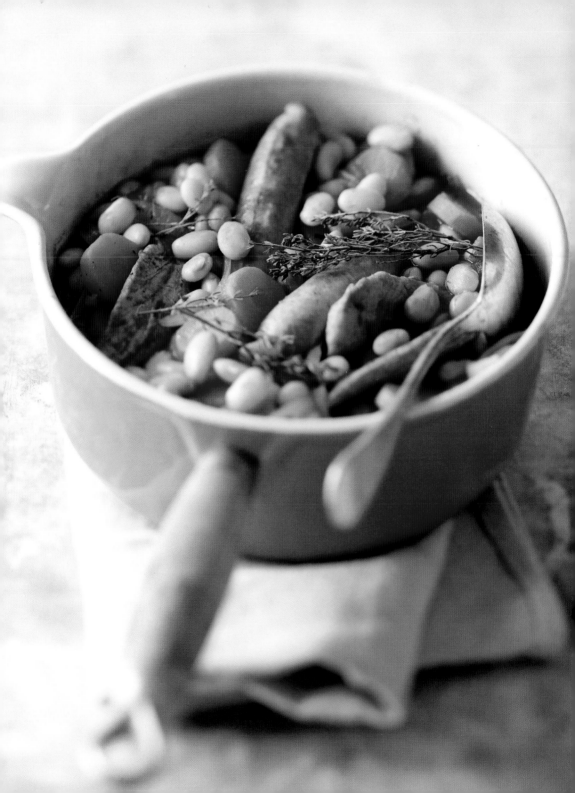

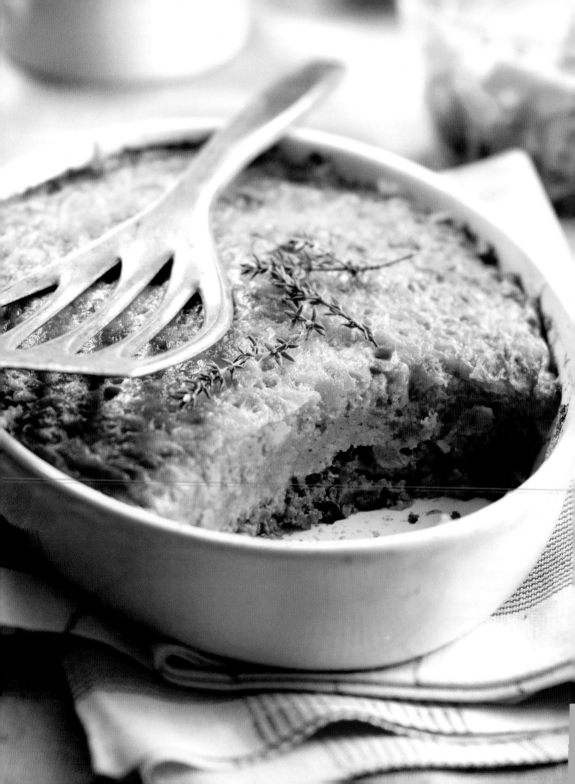

Cottage pie
Hachis Parmentier diététique

This family favorite is usually made from inexpensive mashed potato and leftover ground (minced) meat. To make this one-dish meal more balanced, replace half the mashed potato with puréed vegetables—broccoli, for example. You could also use carrots or zucchini (courgettes) or even a mixture of the two.

PREP TIME 25 minutes | **COOK TIME** 45 minutes

INGREDIENTS FOR 4 PEOPLE

14 oz. (400 g) potatoes

2 onions

1 clove garlic

1 small bunch parsley

14 oz. (400 g) lean ground (minced) beef (5% fat)

7 oz. (200 g) canned tomatoes in juice

2 teaspoons thyme leaves

2 eggs

2 ½ lb. (1.2 kg) broccoli florets
  (to make 1 ¾ lb./800g broccoli purée)

1 teaspoon grated nutmeg

¾ cup (3 ½ oz./100 g) grated
  Swiss cheese

Salt and pepper

1 Preheat the oven to 375°F (190°C/Gas mark 5).

2 Wash and peel the potatoes then steam cook them until tender when pierced with the tip of a knife. Put into a bowl and mash with a fork, without adding any fat.

3 Peel and finely chop the onions and peel and crush the garlic. Wash, dry, and chop the parsley. Dry-fry the onion and garlic in a nonstick skillet (frying pan) until translucent, then add the ground beef. When the meat is browned all over, stir in the tomatoes and a little of their juice, the thyme, and the chopped parsley and cook for 2–3 minutes, then remove from the heat and let cook slightly. Beat and season the eggs then add them to the meat.

4 Boil or steam the broccoli for 5–10 minutes or until very tender, then mash to make a purée, without adding any fat. Mix with the mashed potato. Season with salt, pepper, and the grated nutmeg.

5 Spread out the tomato and meat mixture in the bottom of a gratin dish, then spread over the potato and broccoli mash. Sprinkle over the grated cheese and bake in the oven for about 25 minutes.

6 Serve hot.

Leek *tartiflette*
Tartiflette diététique aux poireaux

In France, where going through the winter months without eating tartiflette would be unthinkable, this low-calorie recipe is a lifesaver for those who've decided to watch their weight. Replacing some of the carbohydrates with leeks makes the dish lighter, of course, but it also makes it richer in fiber, vitamins, and minerals. The traditional whole reblochon cheese has been replaced with cancoillotte, a runny cheese from the Franche-Comté region of France, which is naturally lighter (if unavailable, substitute another low-fat soft cheese). Likewise, using chopped ham rather than bacon makes this dish healthier, lower in calories, and the perfect ally for your skiing vacation!

PREP TIME 30 minutes | **COOK TIME** 45 minutes

INGREDIENTS FOR 4 PEOPLE
14 oz. (400 g) potatoes
1 ¾ lb. (800 g) leeks
8 slices good-quality lean ham
2 onions
1 teaspoon cumin seeds
½ cup (5 ½ oz./160 g) cancoillotte cheese, or other low-fat soft or easy melt cheese
Salt and pepper

1   Preheat the oven to 400°F (200°C/Gas mark 6).

2   Wash the potatoes under running water, then peel them. Steam them for 10 minutes until tender when pierced with the tip of a knife, then cut them into ½-in. (1-cm) thick sticks.

3   Wash the leeks, then finely chop them. Dry-fry them in a nonstick sauté pan over a high heat, stirring constantly, for about 6 minutes until softened. Season with salt and pepper. Set aside.

4   Dice the sliced ham. Peel and chop the onions and dry-fry them until they are transparent.

5   Spread the potato out in the bottom of a gratin dish and season with salt and pepper. Sprinkle with the onions, then cover with the leeks and the diced ham. Sprinkle over the cumin seeds and pour the cancoillotte (if using another soft cheese heat gently until runny enough to pour) over the top. Cook in the oven for 15–20 minutes.

6   Serve straight from the oven.

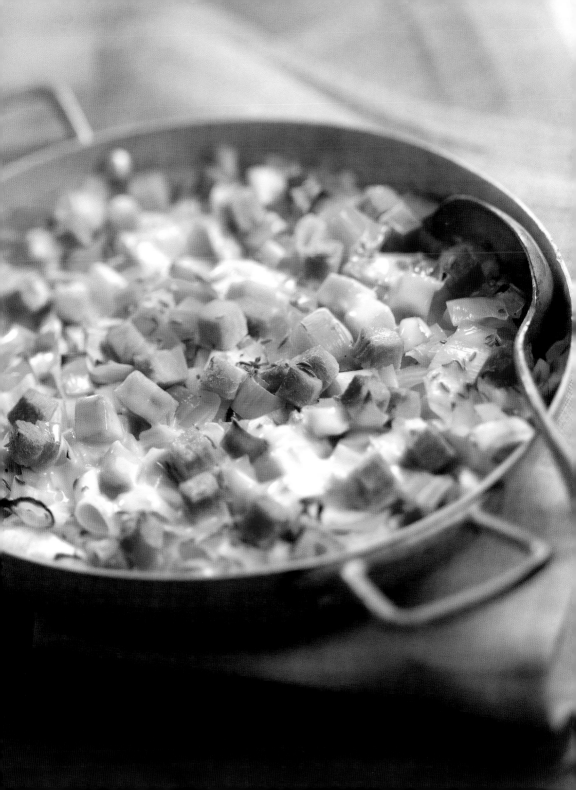

Chicken pot roast
Poule au pot farcie

This traditional French dish is said to date back to the time of Henri IV who, concerned for the welfare of his subjects, is said to have declared, "I want every laborer in my kingdom to be able to put a chicken in the pot on Sundays." Enjoy a lighter version of this famous recipe, with a healthier stuffing.

PREP TIME 45 minutes | **COOK TIME** 2 hours 50 minutes

INGREDIENTS FOR 4 PEOPLE OR MORE

1 onion
1 clove garlic
1 stick celery
1 x 4 ½-lb. (2-kg) chicken with giblets
1 marrowbone
Pinch of grated nutmeg
1 bouquet garni
2 medium (9 oz./250 g) carrots
9 oz. (250 g) turnips
2 leeks, white parts only
4 green cabbage leaves
4 small potatoes
Salt and pepper

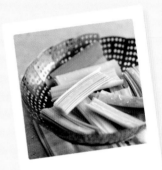

FOR THE STUFFING

3 ½ oz. (100 g) lean smoked
   Canadian-style (back) bacon
2 oz. (60 g) sliced bread
2 tablespoons fat-free milk
1 shallot
2 cloves garlic
1 bunch parsley
1 bunch chervil
4 ½ oz. (125 g) lean ham
1 egg
Salt and pepper

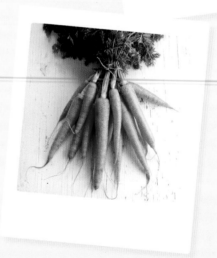

1 Make the stock: peel the onion and garlic, and wash the celery stick. Wash the giblets, set aside the liver, and put the remaining giblets in a large cooking pot with the marrowbone, onion, garlic, celery, nutmeg, and bouquet garni. Add 6 ½ pints (3 liters) water, season with salt and pepper, and simmer for 1 hour.

2 Meanwhile, make the stuffing. Remove and discard the greenish parts of the liver, then wash it and pat it dry with absorbent paper towels. Dry-fry in a nonstick skillet (frying pan) for 3 minutes. Chop the bacon, add it to the pan, and brown for 2 minutes. Set aside. Crumble the bread onto a dish and sprinkle over the milk.

3 Peel the shallot and garlic. Wash and thoroughly dry the parsley and chervil. Finely chop the herbs together with the liver, cooled bacon, and the ham. Add the milk-soaked bread crumbs to this mixture. Beat the egg and stir it in. Season with salt and pepper. Set aside 4 tablespoons of this stuffing and use the remainder to stuff the chicken. Truss the chicken.

4 Peel the carrots and turnips. Wash them and the leeks and cut into thick pieces.

5 When the stock has been simmering for an hour, strain it and pour the liquid back into the pot. Bring the strained stock to a boil and lower the stuffed chicken into the pot. When the liquid returns to a boil, add the carrots, turnips, and leeks. Cover the pot and simmer for 1 ½ hours.

6 Meanwhile, put the cabbage leaves in a dish and cover them with boiling water. Leave to soak for 5 minutes until they have become tender, then drain and let cool. Put a tablespoon of the remaining stuffing on each cabbage leaf, form into a parcel, and secure with kitchen string.

7 Wash and peel the potatoes. After the chicken has been cooking for 1 ½ hours, add the potatoes and the cabbage packages, and cook for an additional 20 minutes.

8 When ready to serve, lift the chicken and the cabbage packages from the broth and remove all the string. Skim any fat from the broth. Serve a piece of chicken to each person with a slice of stuffing, a stuffed cabbage leaf, a potato, and a selection of vegetables.

Turkey with chestnuts
Dinde aux marrons minceur

Anchored in Thanksgiving traditions, turkey with chestnuts is also popular in France at Christmastime. This bird, which is particularly lean, is a judicious alternative to capon or chicken, which are naturally higher in calories because they are fattened. To keep the calorie content of the whole dish down, make a healthy homemade stuffing for it.

PREP TIME 35 minutes | **COOK TIME** 2 hours 40 minutes

INGREDIENTS FOR 4 PEOPLE

5 oz. (150 g) whole natural chestnuts

½ onion

2 shallots

1 clove garlic

⅓ cup (2 ¾ fl oz./80 ml) fat-free milk

1 ¾ oz. (50 g) sliced bread

1 clove

10 ½ oz. (300 g) lean ground (minced) veal

2 tablespoons chopped parsley

1 egg

1 x 6 ½ lb. (3 kg) turkey

Salt and pepper

1 Prepare the chestnuts. Score the flat side with a sharp knife and drop into a large cooking pot of boiling water. Cook for 3–4 minutes then turn off the heat. Take out the chestnuts a few at a time and peel off the skins. Chop finely.

2 Peel and finely chop the onion and shallots and peel and crush the garlic.

3 Pour the milk into a small pan and bring to a boil, then crumble the bread into it. Let cool, then drain and press the bread by hand to remove the excess liquid.

4 In a nonstick skillet (frying pan), sauté the onions, shallots, and garlic with the clove. Tip into a mixing bowl and stir in the ground veal, chopped chestnuts, drained bread crumbs, parsley, beaten egg, salt, and pepper.

5 Preheat the oven to 400°F (200°C/Gas mark 6).

6 Stuff the turkey with this mixture, then tie up the opening firmly. Place the bird in a baking dish, pour over 4 tablespoons of water, then roast in the oven for 2 ½ hours, basting it regularly.

Dauphinois potatoes
Gratin dauphinois léger

This is the perfect accompaniment for any type of meat dish, whether roasted, stewed, or braised. Everyone loves dauphinois potatoes, so make sure you don't miss out. By making this dish with half fat-free milk and half low-fat sour cream, you can welcome it back to the table for everyone to enjoy!

PREP TIME 20 minutes | **COOK TIME** 40 minutes

INGREDIENTS FOR 4 PEOPLE
1 lb. (500 g) waxy potatoes
2 cloves garlic
½ teaspoon grated nutmeg
4 tablespoons low-fat sour cream (crème fraîche)
1 ⅔ cups (13 ½ fl oz./400 ml) fat-free milk
Scant ½ cup (1 ¾ oz./50 g) grated Swiss cheese
Salt and pepper

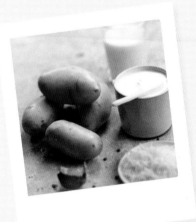

1   Preheat the oven to 300°F (150°C/Gas mark 2).

2   Wash and peel the potatoes. Cut them into thin slices using a mandolin. Peel and crush the garlic.

3   Spread out half the potato slices in the bottom of a gratin dish. Season with salt, pepper, and nutmeg. Sprinkle with half the crushed garlic and drizzle over the sour cream. Lay the rest of the potato slices on top, season, and sprinkle with the remaining garlic. Pour over the milk and sprinkle over the grated Swiss cheese.

4   Bake in the oven for 40 minutes, until the potatoes are tender (check by sticking the point of a knife into them). If necessary, put the dish under the broiler (grill) to brown the cheese.

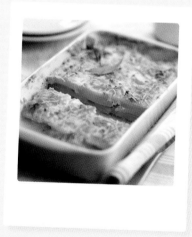

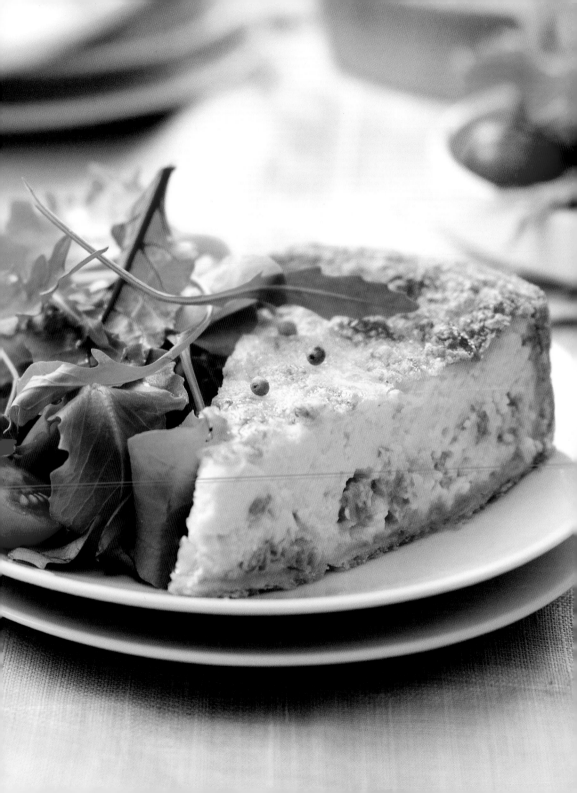

Quiche lorraine

The famous quiche lorraine appears at all sorts of occasions, from a simple lunch at the office to a grand buffet. And everyone adds their own personal touch to it: pie crust (shortcrust pastry) or puff pastry, cream or milk, bacon or ham. Here's another version to try—a light one this time.

PREP TIME 30 minutes | **CHILL TIME** 1 hour | **COOK TIME** 50 minutes

INGREDIENTS FOR 4 PEOPLE
1 onion
3 ½ oz. (100 g) lean smoked
    Canadian-style(back) bacon
2 eggs
Scant 1 cup (7 fl oz./200 ml) fat-free milk
Pinch of grated nutmeg
⅓ cup (1 ½ oz./40 g) grated
    Swiss cheese
Salt and pepper

FOR THE LIGHT PIE CRUST (shortcrust pastry)
Scant 1 ½ cups (6 ½ oz./180 g) all-purpose
    (plain) flour + a little for dusting the work
    surface
Scant ½ cup (3 ½ oz./100 g) nonfat fromage
    blanc or plain nonfat regular or Greek yogurt
1 tablespoon olive oil
3 tablespoons water
2 pinches of salt

1 Make the pie crust by putting the flour, fromage blanc or yogurt, olive oil, water, and salt into the bowl of a food processor. Process until the mixture forms a ball. Wrap the dough in plastic wrap and refrigerate for at least 1 hour.

2 Meanwhile, peel and finely chop the onion and dry-fry in a nonstick skillet (frying pan). Chop the bacon and add it to the pan. Cook until it is golden brown.

3 In a bowl, beat the eggs with the milk. Season with salt, pepper, and nutmeg and refrigerate.

4 Preheat the oven to 350°F (180°C/Gas mark 4).

5 Dust a clean work surface with flour. Remove the dough from the refrigerator and roll it out using a rolling pin. Line a pie plate (tart tin) with parchment (greaseproof) paper and lay the pie crust into it. Bake blind for 10 minutes.

6 Remove the pastry shell from the oven and add the cooked onions and bacon, then pour over the beaten eggs and milk. Sprinkle with the grated Swiss cheese and cook on a low shelf in the oven for 30 minutes. Finish under the broiler (grill) to brown the top if necessary.

Veal Marengo
Veau marengo

This legendary dish, created by the chef Dunand for Bonaparte following the Battle of Marengo, merits a light version. This recipe's secret lies in its low-fat cooking method and the judiciously chosen cut of veal.

PREP TIME 25 minutes | **COOK TIME** 2 hours 45 minutes

INGREDIENTS FOR 4 PEOPLE

1 ¼ lb. (600 g) lean veal fillet

2 onions

1 teaspoon olive oil

2 cloves garlic

⅓ cup (1 ½ oz./40 g) all-purpose (plain) flour

⅔ cup (5 fl oz./150 ml) dry white wine

14 oz. (400 g) canned tomatoes in juice

1 untreated orange

1 sprig thyme

14 oz. (400 g) mushrooms

A few fresh basil leaves

Salt and pepper

1 Cut the meat into large chunks and dry-fry over a high heat in a large nonstick saucepan until golden. Set aside on a plate.

2 Peel and finely chop the onions. Heat the oil in the same pan and sauté the onions until golden. Peel and crush the garlic, add to the pan, and cook for a few minutes until colored. Add the meat, salt and pepper, and flour. Stir to ensure that each piece of meat is well coated in the flour and cook for an additional few minutes. Lower the heat and pour in the white wine. Mix it in well and bring to a boil. Dice the tomatoes and add them, along with their juice, to the pan. Mix well.

3 Wash the orange and remove the zest using a vegetable peeler. Cut in half and squeeze. Add the orange zest and juice and the thyme sprig to the pan and bring to a boil again. Lower the heat and simmer, covered, for 1 ½ hours.

4 Wipe the mushrooms with damp paper towels, remove their stalks, and finely chop the caps. Add to the pan and cook for an additional 15 minutes. Don't forget to remove the thyme sprig and garnish with chopped basil before serving.

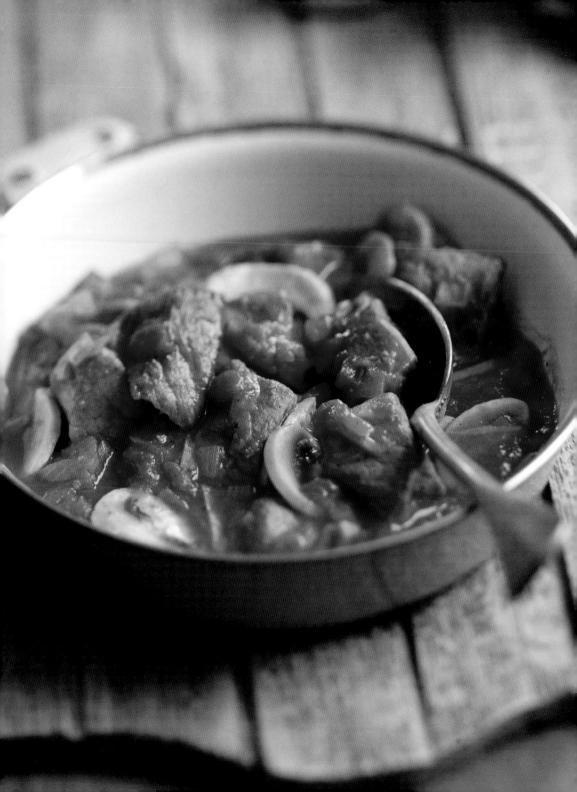

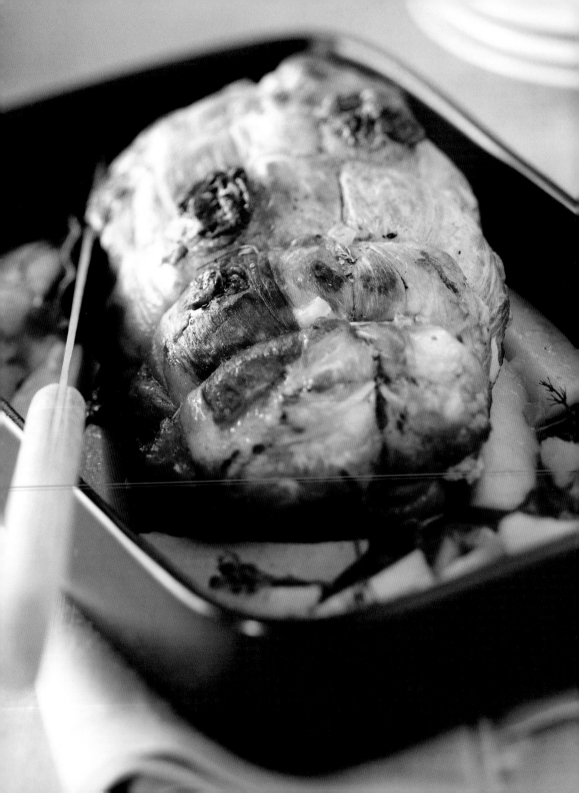

Roast pork stuffed with prunes
Rôti de porc farci aux pruneaux

This classic and tasty recipe is always a great success. So why deny yourself the pleasure of it when dieting? Choose pork tenderloin (fillet) and cook it simply, without adding bacon or fat, for incomparable flavor.

PREP TIME 20 minutes | **COOK TIME** 1 hour 10 minutes

INGREDIENTS FOR 4 PEOPLE
1 ¼ lb. (600 g) pork tenderloin (fillet) roast
4 ¼ oz. (120 g) pitted prunes
1 onion
1 teaspoon olive oil
2 cloves garlic
1 chicken bouillon cube
1 sprig thyme
1 lb. (500 g) potatoes
Salt and pepper

1 Using a sharp knife, make narrow slits in the meat and insert the prunes into the flesh, spacing them apart. Brown the meat on all sides in a nonstick cooking pot, then remove to a plate.

2 Peel and finely chop the onion. Heat the oil in the cooking pot and sauté the onion until golden brown. Peel and crush the garlic cloves, add them to the pot, and cook for a few minutes more.

3 Dissolve the bouillon cube in 2 cups (1 pint/500 ml) boiling water. Return the joint of meat to the pot and add the thyme sprig, stock, salt, and pepper. Simmer for 30 minutes.

4 Wash and peel the potatoes. Cut them in quarters and add them to the cooking pot. Adjust the level of water if necessary and cook for an additional 20 minutes.

5 Just before serving, lift the meat from the pot, slice, and place on a serving plate surrounded by the potatoes. Reserve a ladleful of cooking liquid to pour over the meat and serve hot.

White beans in cream
Mogettes à la crème

Mogettes are a type of white (haricot) bean that is a culinary specialty of the Vendée region, but you can replace them with ordinary dried white beans. Here, the beans are cooked simply with aromatic herbs and spices and served with low-fat cream, for a low-calorie taste of the Poitou-Charentes.

SOAK TIME 12 hours | **PREP TIME** 20 minutes | **COOK TIME** 4 hours 15 minutes

INGREDIENTS FOR 4 PEOPLE
1 ½ cups (10 ½ oz./300 g) dried white (haricot) beans
1 onion
3 cloves
1 carrot
2 sprigs parsley
1 clove garlic
1 sprig thyme
1 bay leaf
Scant 1 cup (7 fl oz./200 ml) low-fat (3% fat) sour cream (crème fraîche)
Pinch of grated nutmeg
Salt

1 Put the dried beans into a terrine dish and cover with cold water. Let soak for 8–12 hours.

2 The following day, drain them, then put them into a cooking pot with ½ glass of water and cook them for 10 minutes over a very low heat.

3 Meanwhile, peel the onion and stick the cloves into it. Peel and wash the carrot. Rinse the parsley. Peel the garlic.

4 Pour 2–4 pints (1–2 liters) water into a large pan and bring to a boil. Put the onion, carrot, thyme, parsley, bay leaf, and garlic into the cooking pot containing the drained beans and cover with boiling water. Cover the pot and simmer over a very low heat for 4 hours. Check and add boiling water as necessary to prevent the beans from drying out. Add salt 30 minutes before the end of the cooking time.

5 When the beans are cooked, add the cream and a pinch of nutmeg. Heat through for 2 minutes. Remove all the aromatics and serve hot.

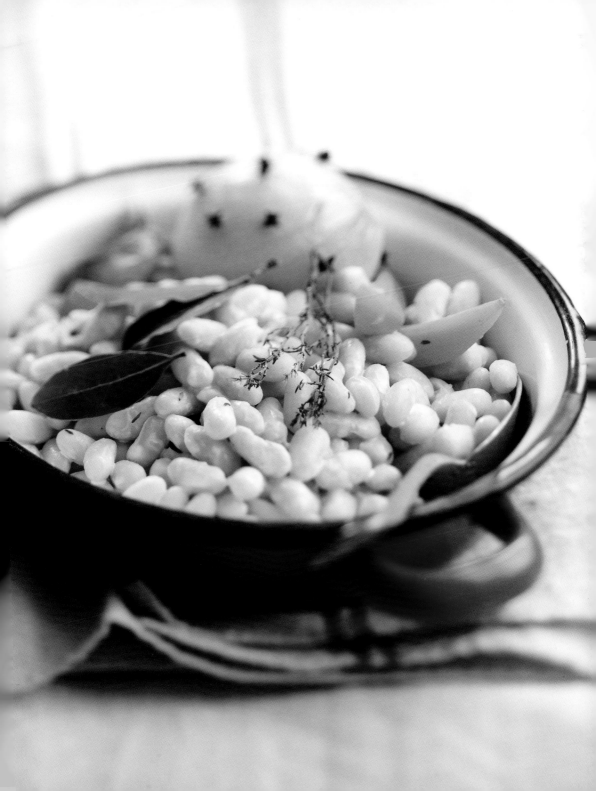

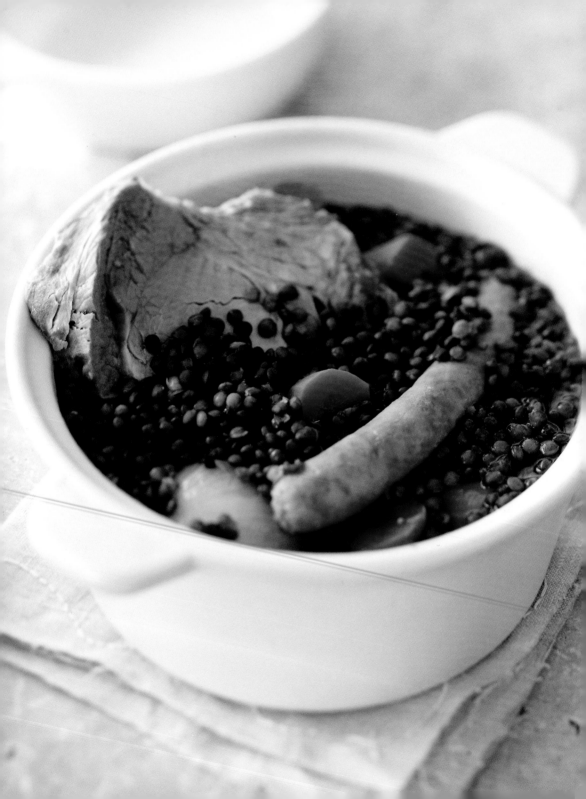

Pork with lentils
Petit salé aux lentilles

The trick for keeping down the calories in this traditional dish lies in the choice of meat. Allow a single chicken sausage (less fatty than pork ones) per person and choose a low-fat cut of pork, removing any visible fat. Everything is cooked together in a pressure cooker with herbs and spices for maximum taste with minimum calories.

SOAK TIME 2 hours | **PREP TIME** 30 minutes | **COOK TIME** 2 hours 30 minutes

INGREDIENTS FOR 4 PEOPLE
1 ½ lb. (650 g) salt-cured lean pork belly
2 carrots
2 large onions
10 cloves
1 bouquet garni
2 cups (14 oz./400 g) Puy lentils
4 chicken sausages
Salt and pepper

1   If your butcher has not given you desalinated meat, soak it for 2 hours in cold water, changing the water a few times. Drain. Using a sharp kitchen knife, remove any visible fat. Put it into a cooking pot, cover with water and season with pepper. Cook over a low heat for 2 hours.

2   Meanwhile, peel the carrots and onions. Stick the cloves into the onions. Put the carrots, onions, bouquet garni, and lentils in a pressure cooker, cover with water, and add a little salt and some pepper. Pressure cook for about 20 minutes.

3   When the meat has finished cooking, remove it from the cooking pot, drain, and cut into large pieces. Prick the sausages with a fork and add to the lentils along with the pork belly. Add 2 glasses of the meat broth for more flavor. Cook, uncovered, over a low heat for 20–30 minutes, checking occasionally to make sure that the lentils don't stick to the pan.

Mini almond pastries
Mini-galettes à la frangipane légère

Various cakes are traditionally served in different parts of France to celebrate Twelfth Night, including galette à la frangipane (puff pastry filled with an almond pastry cream) and brioche with candied (glacé) fruits. The former—the most popular—is a real calorie bomb because of its almond paste filling. As an alternative, we offer these individual pastries with a moist but light filling of apples and almonds. You can slip a (traditional) bean or a trinket in one of them to honor the French tradition of "tirer les rois" (deciding who will be king for the day), if you wish.

PREP TIME 25 minutes | **COOK TIME** 35 minutes

INGREDIENTS FOR 4 PEOPLE
8 ½ oz. (240 g) puff pastry
2 apples
½ vanilla bean (pod)
¼ cup (2 oz./60 g) ricotta cheese
Scant ¾ cup (2 oz./60 g) finely ground blanched almonds
4 teaspoons powdered sweetener for cooking
1 egg yolk

1 Preheat the oven to 400°F (200°C/Gas mark 6).

2 Roll out the pastry using a rolling pin and, using a cookie cutter (or a glass), cut out eight rounds of pastry, each weighing 1 oz. (30 g).

3 Peel and core the apples and cut them into small pieces. Put them into a pan with 2 tablespoons of water. Break open the half vanilla bean and add the seeds to the apples. Cook, covered, over a low heat, then let cool.

4 In a bowl, mix together the ricotta, ground almonds, and sweetener. Divide this mixture between the four pastry rounds, keeping it away from the edges. Spoon the cooled applesauce over the top. Cover with the remaining pastry rounds, sealing the edges with a little water and pressing gently together. Brush with the beaten egg yolk and, if you wish, score the top of the pastry using the prongs of a fork. Bake in the oven for 20 minutes until the pastry is golden.

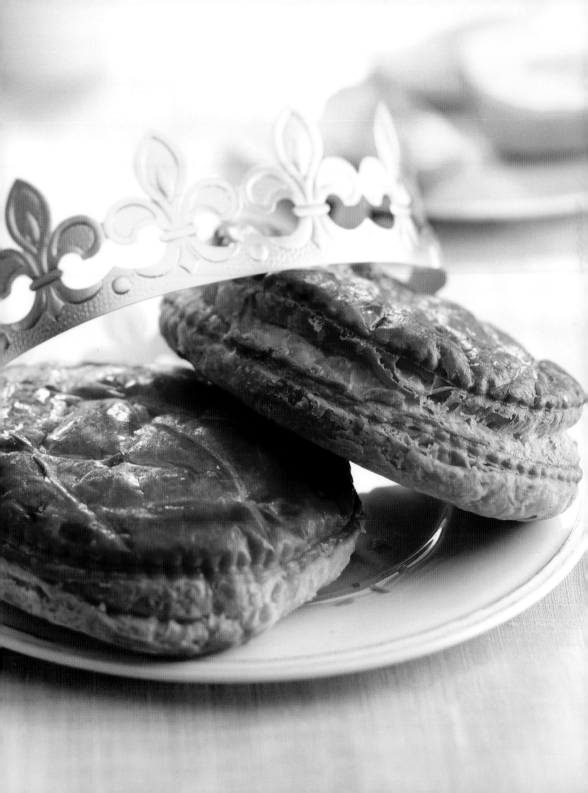

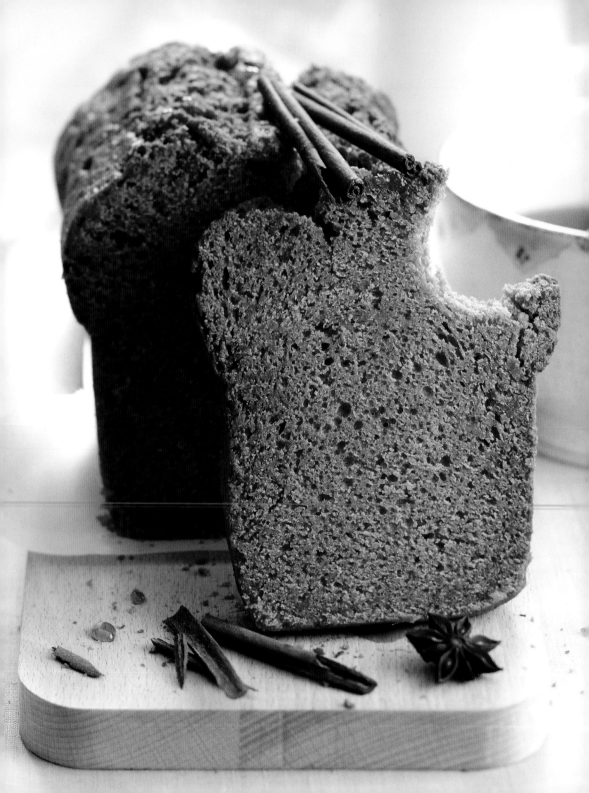

Spiced honey cake
Pain d'épice léger

Pain d'épice is a honey cake flavored with a mixture of spices. Traditionally, it is made with neither eggs nor fat, making it a relatively low-calorie cake. Here, the quantity of honey is halved and the sugar is replaced by sweetener, focusing attention on the spices.

PREP TIME 15 minutes | **COOK TIME** 50 minutes

INGREDIENTS FOR 4 PEOPLE
Scant 1 cup (7 fl oz./200 ml) fat-free milk
⅓ cup (4 ½ oz./125 g) honey
½ vanilla bean (pod)
2 tablespoons powdered sweetener for cooking
Scant 2 cups (9 oz./250 g) all-purpose (plain) flour
1 ½ teaspoons baking powder
1 teaspoon ground star anise
1 teaspoon grated nutmeg
1 teaspoon ground cinnamon
1 teaspoon ground ginger

1 Preheat the oven to 350°F (180°C/Gas mark 4).

2 Heat the milk in a pan with the honey, the seeds from the vanilla bean, and the sweetener.

3 Sift the flour and baking powder into a bowl and stir in the spices, then gradually incorporate the honeyed milk.

4 Pour into a prepared loaf pan and bake in the center of the oven for 45 minutes. Let cool completely in the pan before turning out.

Rum Baba
Baba au rhum léger

Rum Baba is a ring-shaped cake that is soaked in rum-flavored syrup as soon as it is turned out of its mold. It is very often accompanied by sweetened whipped cream (crème Chantilly) and a candied (glacé) cherry, which significantly increases the amount of calories it contains. This is a lighter version of the original: the cake has the same delicious taste spiked with the amber alcohol.

PREP TIME 25 minutes | **COOK TIME** 20 minutes

INGREDIENTS FOR 4 PEOPLE

3 eggs
1 ½ tablespoons (¾ oz./20 g) brown sugar
4 tablespoons powdered sweetener for cooking
Scant 2 cups (9 oz./250 g) all-purpose (plain) flour
1 tablespoon baking powder
2 tablespoons fat-free milk
Pinch of salt

FOR THE SYRUP

4 teaspoons powdered sweetener
  for cooking
½ vanilla bean (pod)
4 tablespoons amber rum

1 Preheat the oven to 350°F (180°C/Gas mark 4).

2 Separate the egg whites from the yolks. In a bowl, whisk the egg yolks with the sugar and sweetener until the mixture pales. Sift in the flour and baking powder, pour in the milk and mix together well using a whisk.

3 Whip the egg whites with a pinch of salt and fold them into the cake batter.

4 Line a ring mold with parchment (greaseproof) paper. Pour the batter into the mold (it should come no more than three quarters of the way up the sides). Bake in the oven for about 20 minutes.

5 Meanwhile, put 1 ½ cups (12 fl. oz./350 ml) of water into a small saucepan with the sweetener and the seeds from the vanilla bean and bring to a boil. Remove from the heat and add the rum.

6 Turn the cake out onto a plate and pour over the rum syrup. Leave it to soak in before serving.

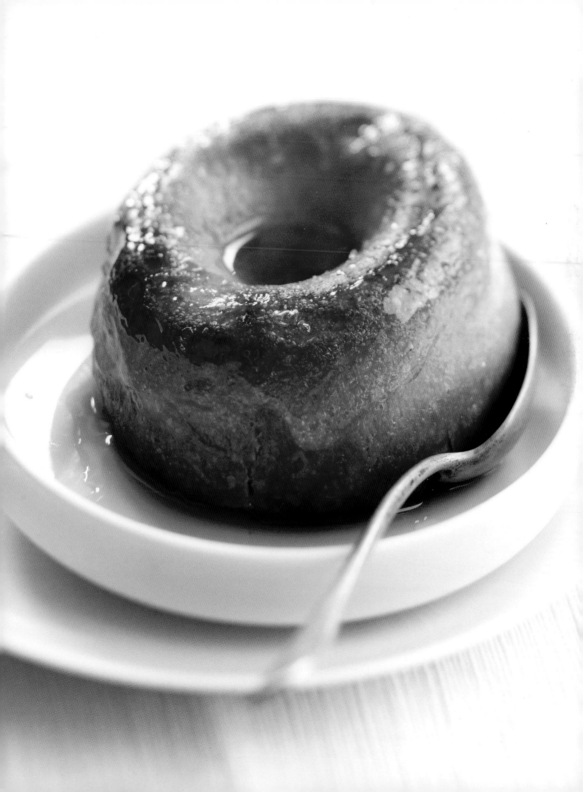

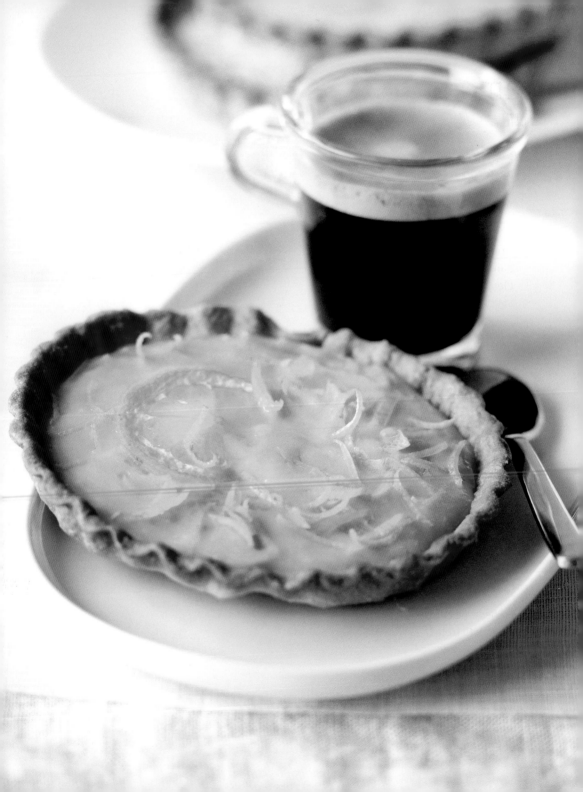

Lemon tart
Tarte au citron allégée

Made of sweetened short pastry with a creamy lemon filling, this tart is a staple of French cuisine. Discover the freshness of this dessert, revisited here with fromage blanc or yogurt, and light, sweetened cream flavored with lemon zest and juice.

PREP TIME 35 minutes | **COOK TIME** 30 minutes | **CHILL TIME** 2 hours

INGREDIENTS FOR 4 PEOPLE
2 untreated lemons
1 leaf (1/16 oz./2 g) gelatin
2 eggs
2 teaspoons (1/3 oz./10 g)
   light butter
2 tablespoons powdered sweetener
   for cooking

FOR THE LIGHT PASTRY
Scant ¾ cup (3oz./90 g) all-purpose (plain) flour
   + a little for dusting the work surface
3 ½ tablespoons (1 ¾ oz./50 g) light butter,
   melted
1 heaped tablespoon nonfat fromage blanc
   or plain nonfat regular or Greek yogurt
2 tablespoons powdered sweetener for cooking
Pinch of salt
2–3 tablespoons water

1   Make the pastry by mixing the flour, butter, fromage blanc or yogurt, sweetener, salt, and 2 tablespoons of water in a mixer or food processor. Check the consistency of the dough and add a little more water if necessary. Process until the mixture forms a ball. Wrap the dough in plastic wrap and refrigerate for at least 1 hour.

2   Remove the zest from one of the lemons using a vegetable peeler. Soak the gelatin in a small bowl of cold water. Squeeze the lemons. Put the lemon juice, eggs, butter, and the sweetener in a saucepan, stir to mix together, and bring to a boil, stirring continually. Remove the pan from the heat, add the drained gelatin leaf and mix in well until it has totally dissolved. Let cool.

3   Preheat the oven to 400°F (200°C/Gas mark 6). Dust a clean work surface with flour. Remove the dough from the refrigerator and roll it out using a rolling pin. Line a pie plate (tart tin) with parchment (greaseproof) paper and lay the pie crust (pastry) into it. Bake blind in the oven for 20 minutes. Let cool.

4   Pour the lemon filling into the pastry shell, sprinkle with the lemon zest, and refrigerate for 1 hour. Serve chilled.

Strawberry tartlets
Tartelettes aux fraises allégées

These pastries made with uncooked fruit enable you to enjoy the pleasures of strawberries while retaining their vitamins, particularly vitamin C. And so that you can enjoy them guilt-free, the pastry is made with light butter and the vanilla cream with fat-free milk. For a pretty effect, arrange the halved strawberries in a rosette.

PREP TIME 40 minutes | **COOK TIME** 35 minutes

INGREDIENTS FOR 4 PEOPLE
1 ¼ cups (10 fl. oz./300 ml) fat-free milk
½ vanilla bean (pod)
2 egg yolks
3 teaspoons powdered sweetener
 for cooking
¼ cup (1 oz./25 g) cornstarch (cornflour)
14 oz. (400 g) strawberries

FOR THE PIE CRUST (shortcrust pastry)
3 tablespoons (1 oz./30 g) cornstarch
 (cornflour)
¼ cup (1 oz./30 g) cake (soft white) flour
2 tablespoons (1 oz./30 g) light
 butter, softened
3 tablespoons water

1 Preheat the oven to 350°F (180°C/Gas mark 4).

2 To make the pastry, put the cornstarch, flour, softened butter, and water into a mixing bowl and mix together using a fork. Form into a ball, turn out onto a clean work surface, and divide into four equal parts. Roll out each piece into a round to fit your individual pie plates (tartlet tins). Line four individual pie plates with parchment (greaseproof) paper and fill with the pastry rounds. Prick the base of the tarts using a fork. Bake blind in the oven for 15 minutes. Let cool.

3 Put the milk and the split and scraped vanilla bean into a saucepan and bring to a boil. Remove from the heat and let infuse. In a bowl, mix together the egg yolks with the sweetener until the mixture pales. Sift in the cornstarch and stir to combine. Remove the vanilla bean from the milk and discard, then pour the milk over the mixture in the bowl, stirring constantly. Return the mixture to the saucepan and heat gently, stirring, until the cream thickens. Pour the vanilla cream into a bowl and let cool.

4 Wash and hull the strawberries and cut them in half lengthwise. Divide the vanilla cream between the four tartlets, then carefully arrange the halved strawberries on top.

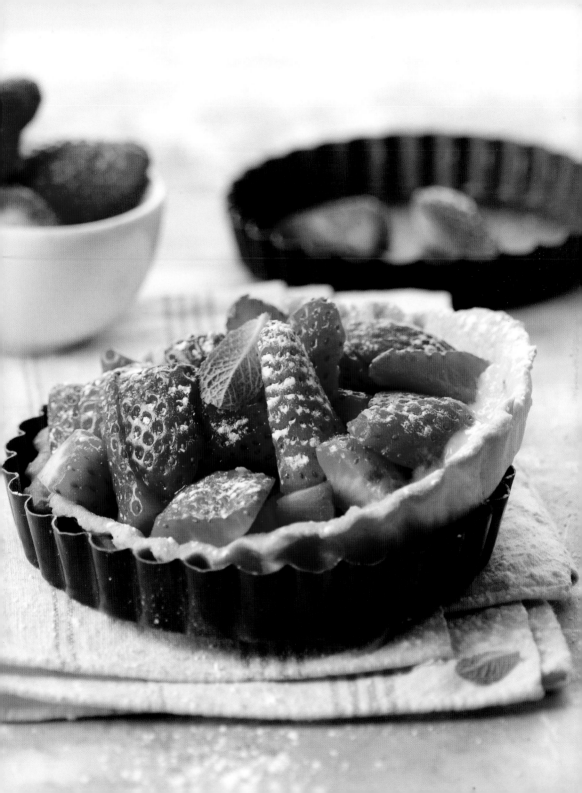

Apple and vanilla profiteroles
Petits choux farcis aux pommes vanillées

Profiteroles, stars of French bistros, are small balls of choux pastry filled with vanilla ice cream and covered with melted chocolate. This variation is filled with vanilla-flavored applesauce and ricotta, a cheese that is low in fat and substitutes perfectly for ice cream.

PREP TIME 40 minutes | **COOK TIME** 45 minutes

INGREDIENTS FOR 4 PEOPLE

4 apples
½ vanilla bean (pod)
¼ cup (1 oz./30 g) cake (soft white) flour
2 tablespoons (1 oz./30 g) cornstarch (cornflour)
Scant 3 tablespoons (1 ½ oz./40 g)
  light butter
5 teaspoons water
Pinch of salt
2 eggs
Scant ½ cup (3 ½ oz./100 g) ricotta cheese
4 teaspoons powdered sweetener
  for cooking
2 oz. (60 g) dark (unsweetened)
  chocolate

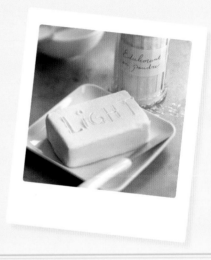

1 Wash and peel the apples and cut them into small pieces. Put them in a pan with a glass of water and the split and scraped vanilla bean. Cover the pan and cook over a low heat until the apple is soft. Remove and discard the vanilla bean and let cool.

2 Preheat the oven to 425°F (220°C/Gas mark 8).

3 Sift the flour and cornstarch into a bowl. Cut the butter into pieces and put into a pan with 5 teaspoons of water and a pinch of salt. Bring to a boil. As soon as it begins to boil, remove the pan from the heat, tip in the sifted flour and cornstarch and mix vigorously using a wooden spoon. The mixture will swell and form a ball that will separate from the pan. If this doesn't happen spontaneously, put the pan back over a low heat and stir until the dough is sufficiently dry to unstick from the pan. Beat the eggs, add half, and mix completely, then add the remainder and mix in. Check the consistency of the dough: it should be fairly firm but supple.

4 Pipe the choux balls (about 8) onto a parchment (greaseproof) paper-covered baking sheet using a plain nozzle in a pastry (piping) bag, or form them using two teaspoons. Space them out on the baking sheet. Cook in the center of the oven for 15–20 minutes. The choux are cooked when they have risen and turned golden brown. Remove them carefully from the baking sheet to cool on a cooling rack.

5 Carefully cut the top off the choux using a serrated knife. In a bowl, mix together the applesauce with the ricotta cheese and sweetener. Fill the choux with this mixture and replace their lids.

6 Break the chocolate into pieces and melt it in a bain-marie with a tablespoon of water. Drizzle the melted chocolate over the choux and serve immediately.

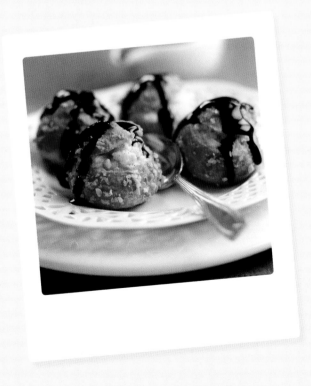

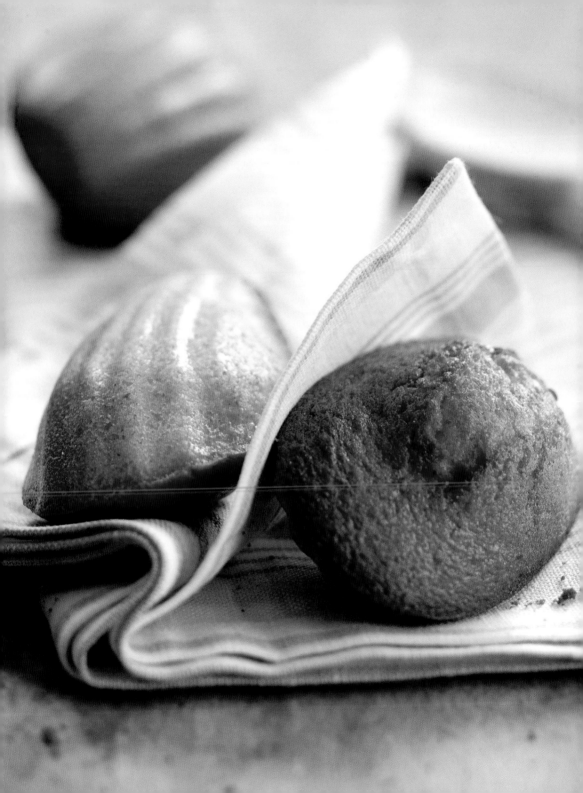

Little lemon madeleines
Petites madeleines légères
aux zestes de citron

A specialty of the Lorraine region of France, madeleines are little shell-shaped cakes. Let yourself be tempted by this light lemon-flavored recipe.

PREP TIME 20 minutes | **REST TIME** 20 minutes | **COOK TIME** 12 minutes

INGREDIENTS FOR 4 PEOPLE
1 egg
4 tablespoons powdered sweetener for cooking
¼ cup (1 oz./30 g) cake (soft white) flour
3 tablespoons (1 oz./30 g) cornstarch (cornflour)
1 ½ teaspoons baking powder
½ untreated lemon
3 tablespoons (1 ½ oz./45 g) light butter, softened

1 In a mixing bowl, beat together the egg and sweetener until the mixture becomes pale. Sift in the flour, cornstarch, and baking powder and fold in.

2 Zest the lemon using a vegetable peeler (or a zester) and stir it into the cake batter along with the softened butter.

3 Lightly oil a madeleine mold using a pastry brush. Using a pastry (piping) bag or a teaspoon, fill the madeleine molds three quarters full with the cake batter. Let rest for 20 minutes. Meanwhile, preheat the oven to 400°F (200°C/Gas mark 6).

4 Bake in the oven for 10–12 minutes. Turn out the madeleines and cool before serving.

Mille-feuilles

Mille-feuilles are pastries that owe their name to the layering of sheets of flaky pastry and cream. Like the original, this recipe is made of puff pastry and crème pâtissière *(French pastry cream), but here the butter is replaced with a leaf of gelatin to enable the layering of the cake, and fat-free milk is chosen over the full-cream variety. Succumb to its marriage of crispiness and creamy vanilla flavors.*

PREP TIME 40 minutes | **COOK TIME** 35 minutes | **CHILL TIME** 30 minutes

INGREDIENTS FOR 4 PEOPLE
10 ½ oz. (300 g) puff pastry (rolled into a rectangular shape)
1 ⅔ cups (13 ½ fl. oz./400 ml) fat-free milk
½ vanilla bean (pod)
1 leaf (¹⁄₁₆ oz./2 g) gelatin
1 egg
3 tablespoons (1 oz./25 g) cornstarch (cornflour)
8 teaspoons powdered sweetener for cooking
2 teaspoons unsweetened light cocoa powder

1 Preheat the oven to 350°F (180°C/Gas mark 4). Cover a baking sheet with parchment (greaseproof) paper. Place the pastry rectangle on top and prick it all over using a fork. Cook in the oven for about 20 minutes until the pastry is golden and dry, then remove from the oven and let cool.

2 Meanwhile, put the milk and the split and scraped vanilla bean into a saucepan and bring to a boil. Soak the leaf of gelatin in a small bowl of cold water for a few minutes. In a mixing bowl, mix together the egg, cornstarch, and half the powdered sweetener. Gradually pour over the boiling milk, continuing to stir. Reduce the heat to low and continue to heat, stirring constantly, until the cream has thickened. Add the drained gelatin and mix well until it has thoroughly dissolved in the cream. Let cool.

3 Cut the puff pastry carefully into 12 equal-size pieces. Spread a puff pastry rectangle with vanilla cream, cover with another piece of pastry, then with more cream, and finally top with another puff pastry rectangle. Repeat to make the other three mille-feuilles.

4 Just before serving, dust each mille-feuille with powdered sweetener and draw zigzags on top in cocoa powder using the neatly cut edge of a piece of parchment (greaseproof) paper as a guide.

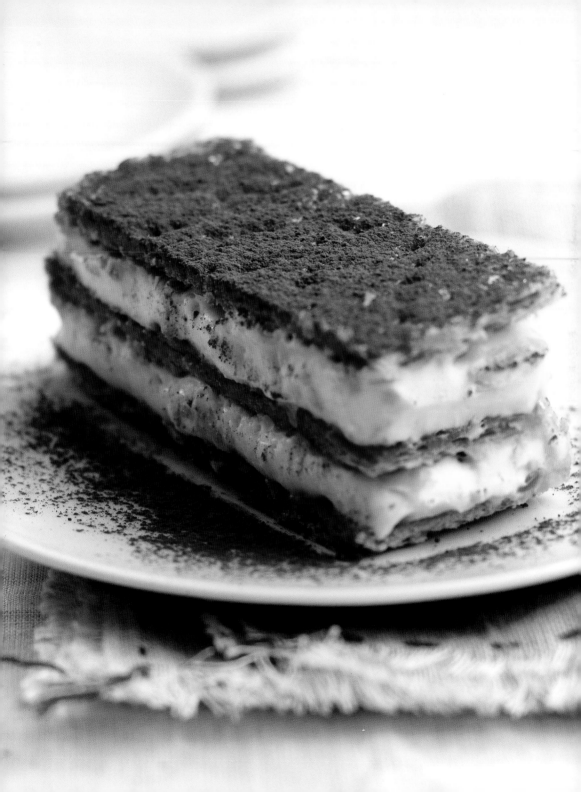

Paris-Brest

Paris-Brest is a French dessert made from choux pastry filled with praline-flavored cream. If you make this recipe with a light choux pastry filled with praline-flavored petits-suisses (French cream cheese from Normandy; if unavailable, substitute fat-free cottage cheese and nonfat Greek yogurt), you'll be free to continue enjoying this traditionally calorie-laden dessert.

PREP TIME 35 minutes | **COOK TIME** 45 minutes | **CHILL TIME** 45 minutes

INGREDIENTS FOR 4 PEOPLE
6 plain nonfat petits-suisses,
   or scant ⅔ cup (5 oz./140 g)
   fat-free cottage cheese + ⅔ cup
   (5 oz./140 g) plain nonfat Greek
   yogurt
1 ½ oz. (40 g) praline
4 teaspoons powdered sweetener
   for cooking

FOR THE LIGHT CHOUX PASTRY
1 tablespoon (½ oz./15 g) cake (soft white) flour
1 tablespoon (½ oz./15 g) cornstarch (cornflour)
4 teaspoons (¾ oz./20 g) light butter
4 tablespoons water
Pinch of salt
1 egg
Generous ⅓ cup (1 ½ oz./40 g) sliced
   (flaked) almonds

1 Preheat the oven to 425°F (220°C/Gas mark 8).

2 Sift the flour and cornstarch into a bowl. Cut the light butter into pieces and put into a pan with the water and salt. Bring to a boil. As soon as it begins to boil, remove the pan from the heat, tip in the sifted flour and cornstarch and mix vigorously using a wooden spoon. The mixture will swell and form a ball that will separate from the pan. If this doesn't happen spontaneously, put the pan back over a low heat and stir until the dough is sufficiently dry to unstick from the pan. Remove the pan from the heat and mix in the egg. The dough should be fairly firm but supple.

3 On a baking sheet covered with parchment (greaseproof) paper, form the choux pastry dough into a ring (of about 8 in./20 cm diameter) using a pastry (piping) bag or two tablespoons. Sprinkle with the sliced almonds. Cook in the center of the oven for 15–20 minutes.

4 Drain the petits-suisses (or cottage cheese) well. In a bowl, stir together the petits-suisses (or cottage cheese and Greek yogurt) and the praline, and add the powdered sweetener. Set aside in the refrigerator.

5 When the choux pastry ring is cooked, remove from the oven and let cool. Once cool, cut it in half horizontally using a pair of kitchen scissors. Fill the bottom half with the praline-flavored cream and top with the almond-coated lid. Chill for 30 minutes before serving.

Waffles
Gaufres allegées

Who can resist a hot waffle in winter when cold, snow, and wind are beating against the windows outside? No one! That's why it's essential to have a light waffle recipe that you can munch on guilt-free—though, of course, you'll need to go easy on the topping, too (a light dusting of confectioner's/icing sugar is much better than a layer of chocolate and hazelnut spread).

PREP TIME 15 minutes | **REST TIME** 1 hour | **COOK TIME** 15 minutes

INGREDIENTS FOR 4 PEOPLE
Scant 2 cups (9 oz./250 g) all-purpose (plain) flour
1 cup (5 oz./150 g) cornstarch (cornflour)
1 tablespoon baking powder
2 tablespoons (1 oz./25 g) sugar
4 tablespoons powdered sweetener for cooking
2 eggs
3 ½ tablespoons (1 ¾ oz./50 g) light butter, melted
Pinch of salt
Scant 1 cup (7 fl. oz./200 ml) fat-free milk

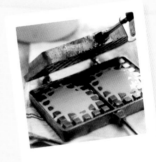

1   In a bowl, mix together the flour, cornstarch, baking powder, sugar, sweetener, eggs, melted butter, and salt. Add the milk a little at a time until the batter is smooth and thick. Cover the bowl with a clean dish cloth (tea towel) and leave to rest for 1 hour.

2   When you are ready to cook the waffles, heat the waffle iron. Spoon a large tablespoonful of batter into the bottom plate of the waffle iron. Close and cook for a few minutes. Repeat until you have used all the batter.

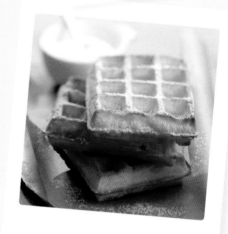

3   Eat while still hot!

183

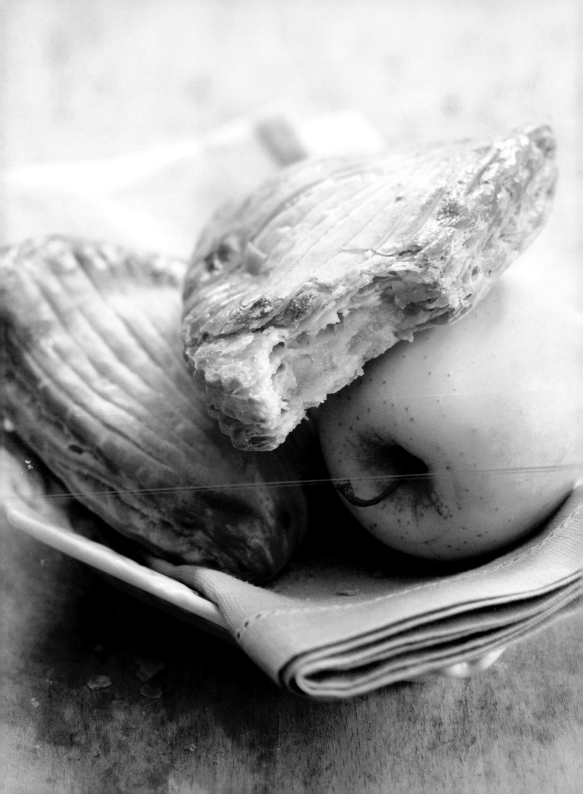

Apple turnovers
Chaussons aux pommes

Leave superfluous calories behind the bakery window and make your own turnovers, for a warm, light, and homemade teatime treat. Their secret? Puff pastry made using petits-suisses (French cream cheese from Normandy; if unavailable, substitute fat-free cottage cheese and nonfat Greek yogurt), filled with unsweetened applesauce.

PREP TIME 35 minutes | **CHILL TIME** 30 minutes | **COOK TIME** 30 minutes

INGREDIENTS FOR 4 TURNOVERS
1 ⅓ cups (10 ½ oz./300 g) unsweetened
    applesauce (purée)
2 apples
1 tablespoon powdered sweetener
    for cooking
1 egg yolk

FOR THE PUFF PASTRY
Scant 2 cups (9 oz./250 g) all-purpose (plain)
    flour + a little for dusting the work surface
1 cup (5 oz./150 g) cornstarch (cornflour)
Pinch of sugar
1 stick (4 oz./120 g) light butter, chilled
8 plain nonfat petits-suisses, or generous ¾ cup
    (7oz./200 g) fat-free cottage cheese + ¾ cup
    (6 oz./175 g) plain nonfat Greek yogurt

1 Preheat the oven to 400°F (200°C/Gas mark 6).

2 Sift the flour and cornstarch into a bowl and stir in the sugar. Make a well in the center. Cut the chilled butter into small pieces. Drain the petits-suisses (or cottage cheese) well. Add the butter and petits-suisses (or cottage cheese and Greek yogurt) to the dry ingredients. Mix the ingredients together using your fingertips until it resembles bread crumbs. Form the dough into two balls, cover with plastic wrap, and refrigerate for at least 30 minutes.

3 Dust the pastry balls and the work surface lightly with flour and roll out the pastry using a rolling pin or a bottle. Cut out eight half moon shapes. Set aside four of them. Prick the other four using a fork, then spread the applesauce over them, keeping clear of the edges.

4 Peel and core the apples then cut them into slices and lay them on top of the applesauce covered pastry. Sprinkle with the sweetener.

5 Cover each semi-circle of pastry with a remaining semi-circle, fold over the edges to seal, then score the top of the pastry using a fork. Beat the egg yolk and brush on the tops of the turnovers. Place the turnovers on a baking sheet and bake in the oven for 30 minutes, turning them over halfway through the cooking time.

Financiers

Although these little teatime treats will never form the basis of a healthy diet, it's always a good idea to reduce calories where you can, and with this light version, you'll be able to eat a second one with a clear conscience!

PREP TIME 25 minutes | **COOK TIME** 30 minutes

INGREDIENTS FOR 4 PEOPLE (8 CAKES)
Scant ⅓ cup (2oz./60 g) brown sugar
8 tablespoons powdered sweetener for cooking
½ cup (4 ½ oz./125 g) finely ground blanched almonds
Generous ⅓ cup (2 oz./60 g) cornstarch (cornflour)
½ cup (2 ¼ oz./65 g) all-purpose (plain) flour
1 stick (4 oz./120 g) light butter
5 egg whites
½ teaspoon powdered vanilla extract, or a few drops liquid extract

1   Preheat the oven to 350°F (180°C/Gas mark 4).

2   In a mixing bowl, mix together the sugar, sweetener, ground almonds, cornstarch, and flour.

3   Melt the butter in a saucepan then let cool.

4   In a separate bowl, whisk the egg whites until they form peaks. Fold them into the dry ingredients, then stir in the melted butter and vanilla extract. Pour the mixture into silicone *financier* molds or mini-muffin pans. Bake in the oven for about 30 minutes. Check the cakes regularly as cooking time varies depending on the oven.

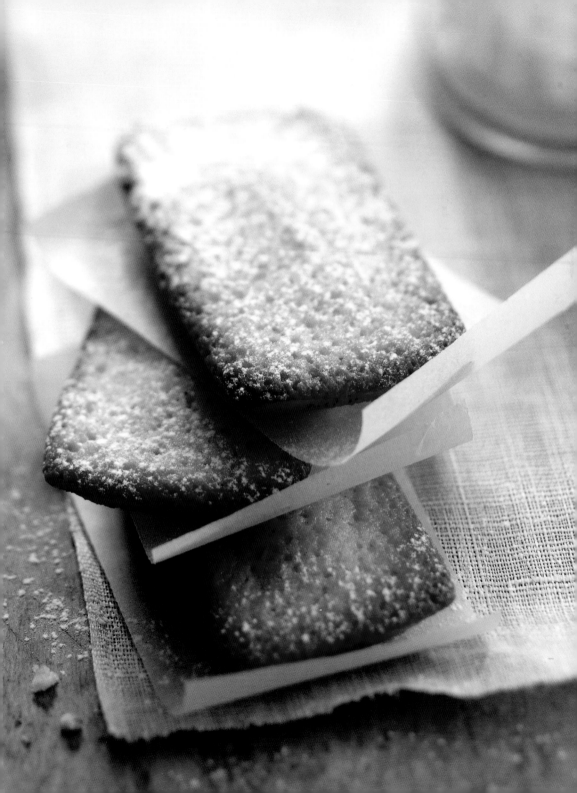

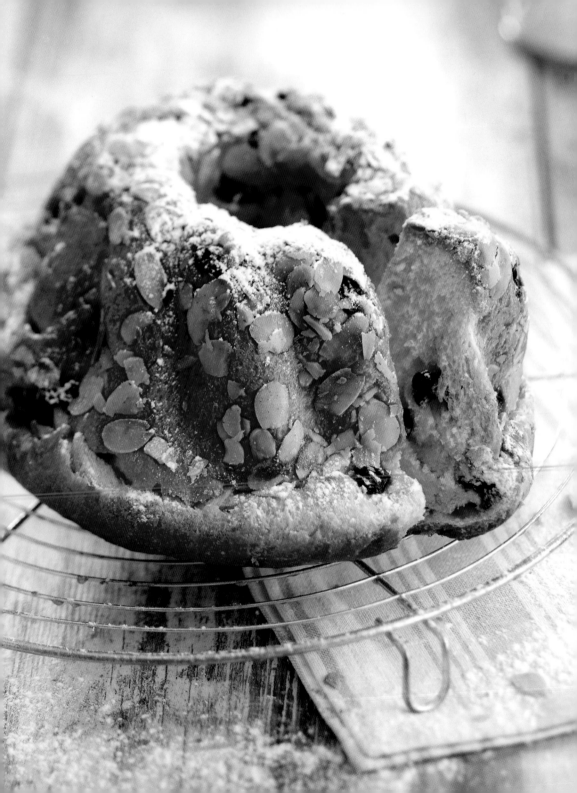

Gugelhupf
Kouglof

This filling cake from Alsace needs lightening up a little as the traditional version is very rich and solid. Our healthier version retains the taste, but has a lighter texture and fewer calories.

PREP TIME 40 minutes | **REST TIME** 1 hour 30 minutes | **COOK TIME** 50 minutes

INGREDIENTS FOR 4 PEOPLE (for a 4-in./10-cm diameter gugelhupf or bundt pan)
¼ cup (1 ½ oz./40 g) raisins
Scant ½ cup (3 ½ fl. oz./100 ml) fat-free milk
½ oz. (12.5 g) fresh baker's yeast
Scant 1 cup (4 ½ oz./125 g) all-purpose (plain) flour
¾ cup + 1 tablespoon (4 ½ oz./125 g) cornstarch (cornflour)
1 teaspoon salt
5 teaspoons (¾ oz./20 g) sugar
4 tablespoons powdered sweetener for cooking
1 egg
⅓ cup (2 ½ oz./75 g) light butter, softened + a little for greasing the mold
2 tablespoons (¾ oz./20 g) whole or sliced (flaked) almonds

1 Soak the raisins in warm water to make them swell.

2 In a saucepan, heat the milk until warm (but not hot). Pour half of it into a small bowl and add the yeast and a little of the flour. Mix to make a paste, then let rest until it has doubled in size.

3 In a bowl, mix the remainder of the flour with the cornstarch, salt, sugar, sweetener, egg, and the remainder of the milk. Knead for 15 minutes to aerate the dough. Add the softened butter and mix in well. Incorporate the yeast; then knead for a few more minutes until the dough pulls away from the side of the bowl.

4 Preheat the oven to 400°F (200°C/Gas mark 6). Lightly butter a gugelhupf (or bundt) pan, making sure you work it into all the grooves. Knock the dough back to its original size by tapping it. Add the drained raisins and mix in well. Put a whole almond into each of the grooves in the mold, then pour the dough into the mold and let rise until it reaches the top. Alternatively, line the grooves of the mold with sliced (flaked) almond. Bake in the oven for 50 minutes. If the cake browns too quickly, cover it with a piece of parchment (greaseproof) paper.

5 Turn the cake out onto a rack and let cool before serving.

Index